Quality Assurance of Aseptic Preparation Services: Standards Handbook

Fifth edition | Parts A & B

Edited by Alison M Beaney
D Prof, MSc, FRPharmS

On behalf of the Royal Pharmaceutical Society
and the NHS Pharmaceutical Quality
Assurance Committee

2016

Quality Assurance of Aseptic Preparation Services: Standards Handbook

Fifth edition

Edited by
Alison M Beaney
D Prof, MSc, FRPharmS
Regional Quality Assurance Specialist North East and North Cumbria
Chair NHS Pharmaceutical Quality Assurance Committee
Visiting Professor, University of Sunderland.

On behalf of the Royal Pharmaceutical Society and the NHS Pharmaceutical Quality
Assurance Committee

© Royal Pharmaceutical Society 2016

First edition published 1993 by the Quality Control Sub-Committee of the
Regional Pharmaceutical Officers Committee
Second edition published 1995 by the NHS QC Committee
Third edition published 2001 by the Pharmaceutical Press
Fourth edition published 2006 by the Pharmaceutical Press
Fifth edition published 2016

Printed in Great Britain by Hobbs the Printers, Totton, Hampshire

ISBN 978 0 85711 307 8

DISCLAIMER

CONTENTS

Acknowledgements, news and updates. Available at: **www.rpharms.com/qaaps**

CONTENTS (CONTINUED)

PART B

Acknowledgements, news and updates. Available at: **www.rpharms.com/qaaps**

QUALITY ASSURANCE OF ASEPTIC PREPARATION SERVICES:
STANDARDS HANDBOOK PARTS A&B

PREFACE

These standards for the quality assurance of aseptic preparation services are a joint initiative between the Royal Pharmaceutical Society and the NHS Pharmaceutical Quality Assurance Committee. We share an aim to develop national standards that support best practice and the care of patients. Pharmacy aseptic preparation services are supporting the care of some of the most critically ill patients.

All the standards have been revised and updated for this fifth edition. The standards are well established and widely used by UK hospital pharmacy departments. Their origin goes back prior to 1993, when the first edition of *Quality Assurance of Aseptic Preparation Services* was published by the NHS Quality Control Sub-Committee.

The relationship between the Royal Pharmaceutical Society and the NHS Pharmaceutical Quality Assurance Committee extends over many years and our publishing division, the Pharmaceutical Press (RPS Publishing), has previously published the third and fourth editions of *Quality Assurance of Aseptic Preparation Services.*

Since 2010 the Royal Pharmaceutical Society has become a body akin to a Royal College. As such, it is appropriate for us to produce and host these standards as part of our library of professional standards. The standards have particular relevance to the RPS leadership roles, including our vision for the pharmacy workforce (RPS 2015).

I would like to join the editor, Dr Alison M Beaney, in thanking the contributors. These standards are a result of the hard work and dedication of many experts from across the UK.

In the UK these nationally agreed quality standards and an audit programme are in place to assure the quality of pharmacy aseptic units (unlicensed) within the NHS. The standards are primarily intended for use within the NHS but they will also be of use to students, licensed units, individuals and organisations in other countries as well as the UK.

[signature]

Ash Soni OBE FFRPS FRPharmS
President Royal Pharmaceutical Society

References

Royal Pharmaceutical Society (RPS) (2015). *Transforming the Pharmacy Workforce in Great Britain: The RPS Vision.* London: Royal Pharmaceutical Society. Available at: **www.rpharms.com/workforce-and-education/transforming-the-pharmacy-workforce-in-gb.asp** (accessed 12 February 2016).

Royal Pharmaceutical Society (RPS). *Quality Assurance of Aseptic Preparation Services* (news). **www.rpharms.com/qaaps**

CHAPTER I INTRODUCTION

Aseptic preparation of medicines is an important part of the service provision by pharmacy departments to facilitate accurate and timely administration of injectable medicines for patients. It is a complex and demanding activity requiring skilled staff, appropriate facilities and close monitoring and control.

Standards to guide and monitor the safe and accurate delivery of these services have evolved gradually, reflecting the changing expectations and needs for maintaining the high quality of aseptic products in the context of rising workload pressures, often reduced resources, and the increasing complexity of modern medicines.

The standards contained herein address these issues in a practical way and should assist both those providing these services and those whose role it is to audit them.

Aseptic preparation in the UK is only exempt from the licensing requirements of the *Medicines Act 1968* and subsequent amendments provided all of the following conditions are met (MCA 1992):

■ The preparation is done by or under the supervision of a pharmacist, who takes full responsibility for the quality of the product

■ The preparation uses closed systems
■ Licensed sterile medicinal products are used as ingredients or the ingredients are manufactured sterile in licensed facilities
■ Products will be allocated a shelf life of no more than one week. The shelf life should be supported by stability data
■ All activities should be in accordance with defined NHS guidelines.

The term 'preparation' is therefore used to denote activity without a manufacturing licence from the Medicines and Healthcare products Regulatory Agency (MHRA), whilst 'manufacture' is used to denote licensed activity.

The first edition of the *Quality Assurance of Aseptic Preparation Services* (Quality Control Sub-Committee 1993) gave advice to ensure consistent quality of products prepared in unlicensed hospital aseptic preparation units. It provided the 'defined National Health Service (NHS) guidelines' required by the then Medicines Control Agency (MCA) in their publication *Guidance to the NHS on the licensing requirements of the Medicines Act 1968* (MCA 1992).

Updated and expanded versions of these guidelines have been published by the NHS Quality Control/Assurance Committee (Lee 1996, Beaney 2001, Beaney 2006). This new edition has similarly been updated and significantly expanded to provide the NHS with up-to-date standards for aseptic preparation.

Since 2006 there have been significant changes to practice that are reflected in this new edition of the *Quality Assurance of Aseptic Preparation Services*. The NHS Pharmaceutical Quality Assurance Committee works closely with MHRA to maintain equity of standards between licensed and unlicensed units. Patients treated with products made in the NHS in either of these types of unit are entitled to expect the same level of safety from the products that they receive.

This fifth edition of the *Quality Assurance of Aseptic Preparation Services* (now published as a standards handbook) includes many new and revised standards in all chapters and places greater emphasis on requirements for pharmaceutical quality systems in EU Good Manufacturing Practice (GMP) (EC 2015) and for quality risk management (ICH 2005). For example, the scope of the Documentation chapter (Chapter 8) has been expanded to reflect this, and the chapter has been renamed. This new edition has been reformatted into two parts: Part A – Standards (contained in the chapters) and Part B – support resources (contained in what were previously termed appendices). In line with EU GMP (EC 2015) the chapters, although standards, use 'should' rather than 'must' throughout. All support resources (which are now published separately) have been revised and updated with the aim of standardising best practice and providing guidance across the NHS on ways of achieving the standards in the chapters. The information in Part B on Computer Validation, for example, has been used as the basis for an advisory document (PQAC 2015) to assist with, amongst other systems, validation of electronic prescribing and so is applicable to an expanded audience.

The standards are applicable to all products prepared aseptically in unlicensed NHS units across the UK for administration to patients. Parenteral nutrition solutions, cytotoxic injections, radiopharmaceuticals and additives for parenteral administration are the most common examples of such products. As such, the products are of a critical nature and standards for their preparation have a significant impact on patient safety. These standards enable pharmacists supervising unlicensed aseptic activity to implement safe systems of work and to prepare products of appropriate quality.

Executive Letter (97)52 (NHS Executive 1997) introduced a requirement in England for regular external audit of all unlicensed aseptic units by Regional Quality Assurance Specialists to ensure appropriate standards were achieved and maintained. This requirement still applies and similar arrangements are in place in the other home countries. The standards in the fourth edition of the *Quality Assurance of Aseptic Preparation Services* (Beaney 2006) are the basis for this ongoing audit programme at the present time, and those in the fifth edition will replace them.

Although *Quality Assurance of Aseptic Preparation Services* is primarily used as the basis of the above audit programme across the UK, the text is also used as standards in several other countries worldwide. Additionally, it is used for undergraduate and postgraduate pharmacy teaching in academia.

The editor, Alison M Beaney, would like to thank all contributors to this edition for their hard work and dedication in preparing these standards. She would like to acknowledge the helpful comments and suggestions received from members of the NHS Pharmaceutical Quality Assurance Committee, the NHS Pharmaceutical Aseptic Services Group, the UK Radiopharmacy Group, the NHS Technical Specialist Education and Training group, and the Medicines and Healthcare products Regulatory Agency.

References

Beaney AM ed. (2001) on behalf of Pharmaceutical Quality Control Committee. *Quality Assurance of Aseptic Preparation Services.* 3rd edn. London: Pharmaceutical Press.

Beaney AM ed. (2006) on behalf of NHS Pharmaceutical Quality Assurance Committee. *Quality Assurance of Aseptic Preparation Services.* 4th edn. London: Pharmaceutical Press.

European Commission (2015). *The rules governing medicinal products in the European Community. Vol IV. Good Manufacturing Practice for medicinal products.* Available at: **http://ec.europa.eu/health/documents/eudralex/vol-4/index_en.htm** (accessed 26 February 2016).

International Conference on Harmonisation of Technical Requirements for Registration of Pharmaceuticals for Human Use (ICH) (2005). *Harmonised Tripartite Guideline, Quality Risk Management, Q9.* Available at: **www.ich.org/fileadmin/Public_Web_Site/ICH_Products/Guidelines/Quality/Q9/Step4/Q9_Guideline.pdf** (accessed 04 April 2016).

Lee MG, ed. (1996). *Quality Assurance of Aseptic Preparation Services.* 2nd edn. Liverpool: NHS Quality Control Committee.

Medicines Act 1968, c67. London: HMSO. Available at: **http://www.legislation.gov.uk/ukpga/1968/67** (accessed 26 February 2016).

Medicines Control Agency (MCA) (1992). *Guidance to the NHS on the Licensing Requirements of the Medicines Act 1968.* London: Medicines Control Agency.

NHS Executive (1997). *Executive Letter (97) 52: Aseptic Dispensing in NHS Hospitals.* London: Department of Health.

NHS Pharmaceutical Quality Assurance Committee (PQAC) (2015). *Computer Systems Validation.* 2nd edn.

Quality Control Sub-Committee of the Regional Pharmaceutical Officers Committee (1993). *The Quality Assurance of Aseptic Preparation Services.* 1st edn. Liverpool: Mersey Regional Health Authority.

CHAPTER 2 DEFINITIONS / GLOSSARY OF TERMS

ACCOUNTABLE PHARMACIST

The pharmacist responsible for all aspects of the services within an aseptic preparation unit. The duties of the Accountable Pharmacist include the approval of all systems of work and documentation used in the unit. This person is also an Authorised Pharmacist.

ACCREDITED PRODUCT APPROVER

An Authorised Pharmacist or a person who has been approved through a nationally recognised accreditation programme for product approval.

ACTION LEVEL

Established microbial or particulate monitoring results requiring immediate follow-up and corrective action. This term is occasionally called an action limit. (BSI 2011).

(BS EN ISO 13408-1:2011 Aseptic processing of health care products – General requirements).

ALERT LEVEL

Established microbial or particulate monitoring results giving early warning of potential drift from normal operating conditions which are not necessarily grounds for definitive corrective action but which could require follow-up investigation. This term is occasionally called alert limit. (BSI 2011).

(BS EN ISO 13408-1:2011 Aseptic processing of health care products – General requirements).

ASEPTIC PROCESSING

Aseptic processing is the manipulation of sterile starting materials and components in such a way that they remain sterile and uncontaminated whilst being prepared for presentation in a form suitable for administration to patients.

ASEPTIC SERVICES VERIFICATION

The process of verifying that the clinical pharmacy verification of the prescription has been carried out, that the prescribed constituents are compatible and the formulation is stable, and that the product is the correct presentation for the intended route of administration.

ASEPTIC WORK SESSION

A period of time where a process or series of processes are performed which can reasonably be expected to present a uniform risk of contamination to the final product(s). Typically a session is the period of continuous work within the aseptic area between breaks and is no longer than a morning or afternoon.

AUTHORISED PHARMACIST

The person designated in writing by the Accountable Pharmacist to supervise the aseptic process and release the product for use.

BIOBURDEN

Population of viable microorganisms on or in the product and/or sterile barrier system. Bioburden is used in aseptic preparation to refer to room surfaces, the surface of items taken into a clean room, product microbial contamination pre filtration or sterilisation. (ISO 2006).

(International Standards Organisation (ISO) Technical Committee (2006). *ISO/TS 11139-1:2006 Sterilisation of health care products – Vocabulary*).

CAMPAIGN BASIS

A campaign basis means that two or more doses may be drawn up from the same vial or the same pool of vials as long as these doses are made sequentially, that no other products are present in the work zone throughout the process, and that the vials stay within the grade A work zone throughout the process.

CHANGE CONTROL

A formal system by which qualified representatives of appropriate disciplines review proposed or actual changes that might affect the validated status of the facilities, systems, equipment or processes. The intent is to determine the need for action that would ensure and document that the system is maintained in a validated state.

CHIEF PHARMACIST

The pharmacist responsible for the pharmacy services within a corporate body. In the context of this handbook, for aseptic facilities not under the direct management control of the chief pharmacist, this responsibility lies with the most senior pharmacist.

CLEAN AIR DEVICE

A clean air device is a piece of equipment that provides a controlled workspace such as horizontal or vertical laminar air flow cabinets, Class II safety cabinets, cytotoxic cabinets, negative and positive pressure isolators.

CLEANING

The removal of organic or inorganic materials from objects or surfaces. This is generally accomplished by a process of wiping using water, detergents or disinfectants. Cleaning is essential before disinfection or sanitisation to remove organic and inorganic materials that may remain on surfaces that potentially interfere with the effectiveness of the process.

CLEAN ROOM

A clean room is a room in which the number and concentration of viable and non-viable airborne particles is controlled. The room is constructed and used in a manner that minimises the introduction, generation and retention of particles inside the room, and other relevant parameters, e.g. temperature and humidity, are controlled as necessary.

CLINICAL PHARMACY VERIFICATION

The process of verifying against the prescription that the product is clinically appropriate for the particular patient.

CLOSED PROCEDURE

A closed procedure is a procedure whereby a sterile pharmaceutical is prepared by transferring sterile ingredients or solutions to a pre-sterilised sealed container, either directly or using a sterile transfer device, without exposing the solution to the external environment.

The use of a solution from a sealed ampoule can be regarded as a closed procedure when a single withdrawal is made from the ampoule, immediately after opening, using a sterile syringe and needle or equivalent device.

The above assumes that, for aseptic preparation and dispensing activities, all closed procedures are performed within a EU GMP Grade A (EC 2015) environment.

CLOSED SYSTEM TRANSFER DEVICE

A drug transfer device that mechanically prohibits the transfer of environmental contamination into the system and the escape of hazardous drug or vapour concentrations outside the system. (NIOSH Alert 2004).

COMMISSIONING

Commissioning is the process of advancing a system from physical completion to an operating condition. It will normally be carried out by specialist commissioning contractors working in conjunction with equipment suppliers. Commissioning will normally be the responsibility of the main contractor. (DH 2007).

COMPONENT

A disposable item that comes into direct contact with the product during preparation.

COMPUTERISED SYSTEM

A set of software and hardware components which together fulfil certain functionalities. For example, the system used to perform parenteral nutrition (PN) labelling may consist of the labelling software, the PC on which the software runs, the server where the database of ingredients is stored and the label printer which produces the final label. It is essential that all of these components work as expected otherwise the desired outcome (a clear, accurate, legible label to put on a product) cannot be achieved.

CONSUMABLE

A disposable item that does not come into contact with the product during preparation.

CONTAMINATION

The presence of viable microorganisms or chemicals, residues and the like (for example dirt and dust) on a surface or within a space.

CONTROLLED WORKSPACE

A controlled workspace is that volume of a clean air device constructed and operated in such a manner and equipped with appropriate air-handling and filtration systems to reduce to a predefined level the introduction, generation and retention of contaminants.

CORRECTIVE AND/OR PREVENTATIVE ACTION (CAPA)

A system that eliminates the cause of a detected deviation or other undesirable situation (corrective action) or the cause of a potential deviation or other undesirable potential situation (preventative action).

CRITICAL ZONE

The critical zone is that part of the controlled workspace where the aseptic manipulation is carried out. Particulate and microbiological contamination should be reduced to levels appropriate to the intended use, normally EU GMP Grade A (EC 2015).

DESIGN QUALIFICATION

The documented verification that the facilities, systems and equipment, as installed or modified, comply with the user requirements specification (URS) and GMP.

DOP

DOP is an abbreviation for Dispersed Oil Particulate and is an aerosol used to test the integrity of high efficiency particulate air (HEPA) filters, usually produced using poly alpha olefin oil.

DETERGENT

A cleaning agent that has wetting and emulsifying properties, used to aid the removal of residues, microorganisms and soiling from a surface.

DISINFECTION

The process of reducing the number of vegetative microorganisms in or on an inanimate matrix by the action of an agent on their structure or metabolism, to a level judged to be appropriate for a specified, defined purpose.

EXTERNAL AUDIT

An external audit is undertaken by staff who are not managerially accountable within the corporate structure in which the aseptic preparation unit is situated, and are independent of any service provision to the unit.

FINGER DAB

A print of 5 digits from a gloved hand on an agar plate. EU GMP (EC2015) uses the term "glove print". (EC 2015).

GASEOUS BIODECONTAMINATION

A sanitisation technique using disinfectants in a vapour phase often used in specially designed isolators. Biodecontamination is the removal of microbiological contamination or its reduction to an acceptable level. There are a number of vapours available for gaseous biodecontamination; the most common is hydrogen peroxide. MHRA refer to these devices as gassed or gassing isolators (MHRA 2015). (ISO 2005).

(International Standards Organisation (ISO) (2005). *ISO 13408-6:2005 Aseptic processing of health care products – Isolator systems*).

GENE THERAPY

Introduction into the human body of genes or cells containing genes foreign to the body for the purposes of treatment, diagnosis or curing disease. (See Part B – 6).

HAND WASH-STATION

A built-in sink used for washing and usually drying hands prior to entry into the clean room.

HIGH EFFICIENCY PARTICULATE AIR (HEPA) FILTER

A filter with classification H13 to H14 when tested according to BS EN 1822-1. H13 filters have an efficiency of 99.95% at most penetrating particle size (mpps). H14 filters have an efficiency of 99.995% at mpps. This does not relate to the DOP test limits. The classification of filters is a factory test using particles of a defined size whereas the DOP test is an in situ test using a range of particle sizes. If replacement H14 filters are ordered for clean rooms operated at EU GMP Grade B (EC 2015), the supplier should be informed that they need to pass the DOP test limit of 0.001% in situ. There is a move to reclassify filters. (BSI 2009).

(British Standards Institute BSI (2009). *BS EN 1822-1:2009 High Efficiency Air Filters (EPA, HEPA and ULPA) – Classification, performance testing, marketing*).

HIGH-RISK PRODUCTS

Those (medicinal) products whose preparation and/or administration in clinical areas have been identified by risk assessment as most likely to pose a significant risk to patients. (NPSA 2007).

HORIZONTAL AUDIT

The most familiar type of audit that examines one element of the standard on more than one item, e.g. documentation.

IMPACT ASSESSMENT

The process of identifying the anticipated or actual impacts of an intervention on those social, economic and environmental factors which the intervention is designed to affect or may inadvertently affect product quality.

INSTALLATION QUALIFICATION (IQ)

The document verification that the facilities, systems and equipment, as installed or modified, comply with the approved design and the manufacturer's recommendations.

INTERNAL AUDIT

An internal audit is undertaken by staff who are a part of the management organisational structure of the department. This is sometimes termed self-inspection.

LINEAR AUDIT

A process whereby the auditor follows the process from beginning to end (trace forward), or in reverse (trace back), if appropriate.

LIQUID BIODECONTAMINATION

A sanitisation technique using liquid disinfectants either impregnated onto wipes or in a spray bottle or canister. When used in combination the process is called spray and wipe. (Cockcroft et al 2001).

LOW-RISK PRODUCTS

Those (medicinal) products whose preparation and/or administration have been identified by risk assessment as least likely to pose a significant risk to patients. (NPSA 2007).

MANAGEMENT REVIEW

A periodic review with the involvement of senior management. A review of the operation of the pharmaceutical quality system to identify the opportunities for continual improvement of products, processes and the system itself to ensure its continuing suitability and effectiveness.

MANUFACTURE (IN RELATION TO CLINICAL TRIALS)

In relation to an Investigational Medicinal Product (IMP), includes any process carried out in the course of making the product but does not include dissolving or dispersing the product in, or diluting it or mixing it with, some other substance used as a vehicle for the purpose of administering it. (*The Medicines for Human Use (Clinical Trials) Regulations 2004*).

OPERATIONAL QUALIFICATION (OQ)

The documented verification that the facilities, systems and equipment, as installed or modified, perform as intended throughout the anticipated operating ranges. Tests should confirm upper and lower operating limits.

PERFORMANCE QUALIFICATION (PQ)

The documented verification that systems and equipment can perform effectively and reproducibly based on the approved process method and product specification.

PHARMACEUTICAL ISOLATOR

A pharmaceutical isolator is a containment device that utilises barrier technology for the enclosure of a controlled workspace for the preparation of aseptic products.

PHARMACEUTICAL ISOLATOR TRANSFER DEVICE (TRANSFER HATCH)

Mechanism to effect movement of material into or out of isolators while minimising ingress or egress of unwanted matter. Isolator transfer devices are often referred to as isolator hatches (MHRA 2015). (BSI 2004).

(BS EN ISO 14644 – 7:2004 Cleanrooms and associated controlled environments. Separative devices (clean air hoods, gloveboxes, isolators and mini-environments)).

PHARMACEUTICAL QUALITY SYSTEM (PQS)

A management system to direct and control pharmaceutical operations with regard to quality. (ICH 2008).

PRIMARY PACKAGING

The packaging that immediately encloses a single unit. In the case of a sterile component the primary packaging will maintain the sterility of the individual unit.

PROCESS VALIDATION (PV)

The documented evidence that the process, operated within established parameters, can perform effectively and reproducibly to produce a medicinal product meeting its predetermined specifications and quality attributes. (EC 2015).

QUALITY REVIEW

An activity that checks whether the Pharmaceutical Quality System (PQS) is capable of achieving its established objectives. The use of Key Performance Indicators (KPIs) for both process, and quality, e.g. number of overdue audit actions, is beneficial, including a regular review with senior management.

READY-TO-ADMINISTER INJECTABLE PRODUCTS

These products require no further dilution or reconstitution and are presented in the final container or device, ready for administration or connection to a needle or administration set, e.g. an infusion in a bag with no additive required. (NPSA 2007).

READY-TO-USE INJECTABLE PRODUCTS

These products require no further dilution or reconstitution before transfer to an administration device; for example, a liquid within an ampoule or vial, of the required concentration, that only needs to be drawn up into a syringe. (NPSA 2007).

RECOMMISSIONING

The process of repeating the commissioning tests for a specific facility at a defined frequency to demonstrate continued compliance with operating conditions. This is often carried out immediately after servicing a piece of equipment.

RISK

The combination of the probability (likelihood) of occurrence of harm and the severity (consequence) of that harm (based on ISO/IEC Guide 51) (ISO 2014). (ICH 2005).

RISK ACCEPTANCE

The decision to accept risk (ISO Guide 73) (ISO 2009). (ICH 2005).

RISK ANALYSIS

The estimation of the risk associated with the identified hazards. (ICH 2005).

RISK ASSESSMENT

A systematic process of organising information to support a risk decision to be made within a risk management process. It consists of the identification of hazards and the analysis and evaluation of risks associated with exposure to those hazards. (ICH 2005).

RISK COMMUNICATION

The sharing of information about risk and risk management between the decision maker and other stakeholders. (ICH 2005).

RISK CONTROL

Actions implementing risk management decisions (ISO Guide 73) (ISO 2009). (ICH 2005).

RISK EVALUATION

The comparison of the estimated risk to given risk criteria using a quantitative or qualitative scale to determine the significance of the risk. (ICH 2005).

RISK IDENTIFICATION

The systematic use of information to identify potential sources of harm (hazards) referring to the risk question or problem description. (ICH 2005).

RISK MANAGEMENT

The systematic application of quality management policies, procedures, and practices to the tasks of assessing, controlling, communicating and reviewing risk. (ICH 2005).

RISK REDUCTION

Actions taken to lessen the probability of occurrence of harm and the severity of that harm. (ICH 2005).

RISK REVIEW

Review or monitoring of output/results of the risk management process considering (if appropriate) new knowledge and experience about the risk. (ICH 2005).

SANITISATION

Sanitisation is the process of achieving pharmaceutically clean objects and surfaces by cleaning and disinfection processes.

SECONDARY PACKAGING

The packaging that encloses multiples of individual units. The secondary packaging may be removed without affecting the characteristics of the product, e.g. loss of sterility.

In the context in which the term is used in this handbook, any packaging that encloses, for example, a single ampoule or vial is considered to be secondary packaging.

SHORT-TERM USE

Products for short-term use should commence administration within 24 hours of preparation on condition that stability data is satisfactory. They will have been prepared under controlled conditions complying with the guidance in Part B – 4.

SPORICIDE

A chemical that can penetrate the outer wall of a spore and kill the microorganism.

STANDARD OPERATING PROCEDURES

Standard operating procedures are detailed written documents formally approved by the Accountable Pharmacist. They describe the operations to be carried out, the precautions to be taken and the measures to be applied that are directly or indirectly related to the preparation and supply of the product. They give directions for performing certain operations, e.g. cleaning, changing, environmental monitoring and equipment operation, to ensure that they are performed to a consistent standard.

STARTING MATERIAL (INGREDIENT)

Any substance used in the preparation of a medicinal product, excluding components and consumables.

STERILITY ASSURANCE LEVEL

Sterility assurance level (SAL) is the probability that a process makes something sterile. A sterilisation process must deliver a SAL of 1 in a million (10^{-6}).

STERILISATION

Sterilisation is the process of killing all microorganisms present. It is an absolute term.

SUPPORT ROOM

The support room is a dedicated room that is used for activities that are ancillary to the aseptic preparation process. Such activities may include component assembly, generation of documentation, labelling, checking and packaging.

Note: The support room may be known by other terms, e.g. preparation room, layup room, collation room and there may be more than one, i.e. inner and outer support rooms.

USER REQUIREMENTS SPECIFICATION (URS)

The set of owner, user and engineering requirements necessary and sufficient to create a feasible design, meeting the intended purpose of the system.

VALIDATION

The accumulation of documentary evidence to show that a system, equipment or process will consistently perform as expected to a predetermined specification, and will continue to do so throughout its life cycle.

It establishes documented evidence which provides a high degree of assurance that a specific process will consistently produce a product meeting its predetermined specifications and quality attributes.

VALIDATION MASTER PLAN (VMP)

A co-ordinating document describing the validation of a total system comprising individual pieces of equipment and/or process.

The VMP should begin with policy and strategy for total system validation and show how different items of equipment and processes are to interact to form a total system. It should list all associated validation documents, including individual validation plans and protocols, and should include those documents in existence and those to be created to complete the validation study.

References

British Standards Institute (BSI) (2004). *BS EN ISO 14644 – 7:2004. Cleanrooms and associated controlled environments. Separative devices (clean air hoods, gloveboxes, isolators and mini-environments).* London: BSI.

British Standards Institute (BSI) (2009). *BS EN 1822-1:2009 High Efficiency Air Filters (EPA, HEPA and ULPA) – Classification, performance testing, marketing.* London: BSI.

British Standards Institute (BSI) (2011). *BS EN ISO 13408-1:2011 Aseptic processing of health care products - General requirements.* London: BSI.

Cockcroft MG et al (2001). Validation of liquid disinfection techniques for transfer of components into hospital pharmacy clean rooms. *Hospital Pharmacy* 8: 226-232.

Department of Health (DH) (2007). *Specialised ventilation for healthcare premises.* Health Technical Memorandum 03-01:2007. London: Department of Health.

European Commission (EC) (2015). *The rules governing medicinal products in the European Community. Vol IV. Good Manufacturing Practice for medicinal products.* Available at: ***http://ec.europa.eu/health/documents/eudralex/vol-4/index_en.htm*** (accessed 26 February 2016).

Note: the detailed guidelines of EU GMP (EC 2015) are also set out in:

Medicines and Healthcare products Regulatory Agency (MHRA). *Rules and Guidance for Pharmaceutical Manufacturers and Distributors.* Current edn. London: Pharmaceutical Press.

International Conference on Harmonisation of Technical Requirements for Registration of Pharmaceuticals for Human Use (ICH) (2005). *Harmonised Tripartite Guideline, Quality Risk Management, Q9.* Available at: ***www.ich.org/fileadmin/Public_Web_Site/ICH_Products/Guidelines/Quality/Q9/Step4/Q9_Guideline.pdf*** (accessed 04 April 2016)

International Conference on Harmonisation of Technical Requirements for Registration of Pharmaceuticals for Human Use (ICH) (2008). *Harmonised Tripartite Guideline, Pharmaceutical Quality System, Q10.*

International Standards Organisation (ISO) (2005). *ISO 13408-6:2005 Aseptic processing of health care products - Isolator systems.* Geneva: ISO.

International Standards Organisation (ISO) Technical Committee (2006). *ISO/TS 11139-1:2006 Sterilisation of health care products – Vocabulary.* Geneva: ISO.

International Standards Organisation (ISO) (2009). *ISO Guide 73:2009 Risk Management – Vocabulary.* Geneva: ISO.

International Standards Organisation (ISO) (2014). *ISO/IEC Guide 51:2014 Safety aspects – Guidelines for their inclusion in ISO standards.* Geneva: ISO.

Medicines and Healthcare products Regulatory Agency (MHRA) (2015). *Questions and Answers for Specials Manufacturers.* London: MHRA. Available at: ***www.gov.uk/government/publications/guidance-for-specials-manufacturers*** (accessed 19 February 2016).

National Institute for Occupational Safety and Health (NIOSH) (2004). *Preventing Occupational Exposures to Antineoplastic And Other Hazardous Drugs in Healthcare Settings.* Available at: ***www.cdc.gov/niosh/docs/2004-165*** (accessed 25 April 2016).

National Patient Safety Agency (NPSA) (2007). *Patient Safety Alert. Promoting safer use of injectable medicines.* NPSA/2007/20. London: National Patient Safety Agency.

The Medicines for Human Use (Clinical Trials) Regulations 2004. SI 2004 No.1031. London: The Stationery Office.

CHAPTER 3 MINIMISING RISK WITH INJECTABLE MEDICINES

Risks to patients are greater when injectable medicines are prepared in clinical areas, such as wards and operating theatres, than when they are prepared in pharmacy under appropriate standards (Austin and Elia 2009). Risks of medication errors and microbiological contamination have been well documented (Crowley et al 2004, Argo et al 2000). Instances of harm to patients continue to be reported, however (NHS England 2013).

Standards for aseptic preparation in pharmacy are clearly defined in this text and others across Europe (EC GMP 2015, PIC/S 2014).

Ideally all injectable medicines should be prepared in pharmacy under these defined and inspected standards (NHS Executive 1997). Unfortunately, however, aseptic capacity within pharmacy to prepare medicines in ready-to-use or ideally ready-to-administer form, is limited. As a consequence, the majority of "aseptic" manipulation is carried out in clinical areas where environmental standards and preparation practices are variable (Beaney and Goode 2003) and risks of medication errors and microbiological contamination exist (Austin and Elia 2009).

A survey on quality assurance standards for preparation across the EU (Scheepers 2010) also showed a gap in standards between pharmacy and ward preparation.

There should be a risk management system across the organisation to minimise risks to patients from injectable medicines (ICH 2005). This involves the following components:

- Risk assessment
- Risk reduction and control
- Risk acceptance and communication
- Risk review.

The use of a risk assessment tool is recommended to identify high-risk products being prepared in clinical areas to target them for pharmacy preparation. A risk assessment tool was developed (Beaney et al 2005) which became the basis of a Patient Safety Alert (NPSA 2007) requiring risk assessment of practices and individual injectable products prepared in clinical areas. There is an ongoing requirement to audit injectable medicines practices in clinical areas (NPSA 2007). Additionally, NHS England created a list of serious preventable patient safety incidents that should never occur (NHS England 2013).

One of these stated that a patient should not come to severe harm as a result of a wrongly-prepared high-risk injectable medicine. This required hospitals to use the NPSA risk assessment tool (NPSA 2007) to identify their own list of high-risk medicines. (A list has been published by the NHS Pharmaceutical Aseptic Services Group (PASG) and UK Medicines Information (UKMI), and is available on their websites. This may be helpful as a basis for a hospital's own list.) Risk assessment allows prioritisation of products of higher risk for pharmacy preparation to make best use of the limited capacity in pharmacy aseptic units.

The EU survey on quality assurance standards for preparation (Scheepers 2010) led to a Council of Europe Resolution, CM/ResAP(2011)1 (EC 2011) which requires risk assessment for aseptic products. This risk assessment mentions similar risk factors to those identified in earlier UK publications (Beaney and Goode 2003, Beaney et al 2005, NPSA 2007). The Resolution CM/ResAP(2011)1 (EC 2011) also states that high-risk products should be prepared in pharmacy, but that low-risk products can be prepared in clinical areas. Further advice is available to assist organisations with these decisions (Scheepers et al 2015).

Even for low-risk products, pharmacy has a role to play in the training of nurses to raise awareness of the risks to patients from preparation and to give advice on "non-touch" techniques (Beaney et al 2005, Beaney and Black 2012). Other risk reduction measures for example, the provision of dose calculation tools or step-by-step preparation methods, can also reduce risks to patients from preparation in clinical areas.

MANAGEMENT OF THE RISKS

3.1   Risk assessment

3.1.1   There should be an up-to-date injectable medicines policy across the organisation defining roles and responsibilities and multi-disciplinary management arrangements.

3.1.2   Risk assessments and option appraisals for the site of preparation i.e. pharmacy or clinical areas, should be performed and documented for preparation of all injectable medicines within the organisation.

3.1.3   The location of all aseptic preparation should be appropriate in relation to the level of risk as determined by use of the risk assessment tool (NPSA 2007). There should be evidence of pharmacy involvement in this process.

3.1.4   An up-to-date list of high-risk injectable medicines for the specific hospital should be maintained reflecting the local situation. Best practice is that a list of NPSA 20 risk ratings should be available for all injectable medicines prepared in clinical areas.

3.1.5   There should be a system for evaluating risks for injectable medicines before they are introduced to the organisation, for example by assessment by drug and therapeutics or formulary committees.

3.2   Risk reduction and control

3.2.1   There should be a pharmacy strategy to effectively manage risks associated with injectable medicines wherever they are prepared (pharmacy, outsourced, or in clinical areas). Pharmacy support should be provided to clinical areas to reduce risks to patients from preparation in those locations. This should be defined in the injectable medicines policy.

3.2.2   An appropriate pharmacy aseptic product list (catalogue) should be maintained and updated regularly. This should include all aseptic products supplied from pharmacy (either prepared in-house or outsourced). This catalogue should be available in all clinical areas to ensure products are not inappropriately prepared there.

3.2.3   Robust arrangements should be in place to specify and monitor the quality of any outsourced aseptic products (see Part B – 3).

3.2.4 Additions to parenteral nutrition solutions (aqueous or lipid phase) contained in infusion bags and/or syringes should only be made in a pharmacy aseptic unit (DH 2011).

3.2.5 Arrangements should be in place for the provision of parenteral nutrition when the pharmacy aseptic unit is closed. Ward-based preparation or additional manipulation of parenteral nutrition components should not occur (DH 2011).

3.2.6 Arrangements for the preparation of intrathecal chemotherapy should comply with national guidance (DH 2008).

3.2.7 Arrangements for intrathecal chemotherapy should comply with Patient Safety Alert NHS/PSA/D/2014/002 (NHS England 2014).

3.2.8 Arrangements for the handling of concentrated potassium chloride solutions should comply with NPSA requirements (NPSA 2002). Ready-to-administer products should be provided to clinical areas wherever possible.

3.2.9 Preparation should use closed systems. An MHRA licence is required for open systems (MCA 1992).

3.2.10 For unlicensed units, the expiry period allocated should not exceed one week (MCA 1992). The shortest practical expiry period should, however, be allocated to minimise the time between preparation and administration and thereby reduce the risk of any microbial contamination multiplying and of chemical degradation (see Chapter 6: Formulation, stability and shelf life). The shelf lives of products should be appropriate and consider microbiological risk as well as physico-chemical stability.

3.3 Risk acceptance and communication

3.3.1 Any residual risks relating to injectable medicines that have not been appropriately controlled as described above should be accepted by the organisation, e.g. by recognising them on the risk register.

3.3.2 There should be a system for communicating decisions about which products are to be made by aseptic units and which can be made in clinical areas so all are aware of their responsibilities.

3.3.3 There should be an effective process in place to communicate any heightened risks, e.g. invoking of contingency plans.

3.4 Risk review

3.4.1 All risks (including risk register entries) should be regularly reviewed at defined time intervals and risk ratings updated as appropriate.

3.4.2 There should be a system to review any errors or incidents in relation to injectable medicines across the organisation and put risk reduction and control measures in place in response to these.

3.4.3 There should also be a system to learn from these type of events that occur external to the organisation and for responding to alerts from national bodies e.g. patient safety bodies.

References

Argo AL et al (2000). The ten most common lethal medication errors in hospital patients. *Hosp Pharm* 35: 470-475.

Austin P, Elia M (2009). A systematic review and meta-analysis of the risk of microbial contamination of aseptically prepared doses in different environments. *J Pharm Pharmaceut Sci* 12(2) 233-242. Available at: **www.cspsCanada.org**

Beaney AM, Goode J (2003). A risk assessment of the ward-based preparation of parenteral medicines. *Hosp Pharm* 10(7): 306-308.

Beaney AM, et al (2005). Development of a risk assessment tool to improve the safety of patients receiving intravenous medication. *Hosp Pharm* 12: 150-154.

Beaney AM, Black A (2012). Preparing Injectable Medicines Safely. *Nursing Times* 108(3): 20-23.

Crowley C et al (2004). Describing the frequency of iv medication preparation and administration errors. *Hosp Pharm* 11: 330-336.

Department of Health (DH) (2008). *Updated National Guidance on Safe Administration of Intrathecal Chemotherapy.* HSC 2008/001. London: Department of Health.

Department of Health (DH) (2011). *Improving practice and reducing risk in the provision of parenteral nutrition for neonates and children.* Report from the Paediatric Chief Pharmacists Group. London: Department of Health. Available at: **www.rpharms.com** (accessed 04 April 2016).

European Commission (2011). Resolution CM/ResAP (2011)1 on quality and safety assurance requirements for medicinal products prepared in pharmacies for the special needs of patients. (Adopted by the Committee of Ministers on 19 January 2011).

European Commission (2015). *The rules governing medicinal products in the European Community. Vol IV. Good Manufacturing Practice for medicinal products.* Available at: **http://ec.europa.eu/health/documents/eudralex/vol-4/index_en.htm** (accessed 26 February 2016).

International Conference on Harmonisation of Technical Requirements for Registration of Pharmaceuticals for Human Use (ICH) (2005). *Harmonised Tripartite Guideline, Quality Risk Management, Q9.* Available at: **www.ich.org/fileadmin/Public_Web_Site/ICH_Products/Guidelines/Quality/Q9/Step4/Q9_Guideline.pdf** (accessed 04 April 2016)

Medicines Control Agency (MCA) (1992). *Guidance to the NHS on the Licensing Requirements of the Medicines Act 1968.* London: Medicines Control Agency.

National Patient Safety Agency (2002). *Patient Safety Alert. Potassium chloride concentrate solutions.* London: National Patient Safety Agency.

National Patient Safety Agency (2007). *Patient Safety Alert. Promoting safer use of injectable medicines.* NPSA/2007/20. London: National Patient Safety Agency.

NHS England (2013). *Never Events data summary for 2012/13.* Available at: **www.england.nhs.uk/wp-content/uploads/2013/12/nev-ev-data-sum-1213.pdf** (accessed 04 February 2016). **www.england.nhs.uk/patientsafety/never-events/ne-data/** (accessed 04 February 2016).

NHS England (2014). *Patient Safety Alert. Non-Luer spinal (intrathecal) devices for chemotherapy.* NHS/PSA/D/2014/002. Available at: **http://www.england.nhs.uk/wp-content/uploads/2014/02/non-Luer-spinal-alert.pdf** (accessed 04 February 2016).

NHS Executive (1997). *Executive Letter (97) 52: Aseptic Dispensing in NHS Hospitals.* London: Department of Health.

PIC/S Secretariat (2014). *A guide to good practices for the preparation of medicinal products in healthcare establishments.* PE 010-4. Geneva: PIC/S Secretariat.

Scheepers HPA et al (2010). Abridged Survey Report on Quality and Safety Assurance Standards for the Preparation of Medicinal Products in Pharmacies. *Pharmeuropa* Vol 22(No 4): 405-413

Scheepers HPA et al (2015). Aseptic preparation of parenteral medicinal products in healthcare establishments in Europe. *Eur J of Hosp Pharm* [online]. Available at: **http://ejhp.bmj.com/content/23/1/50.abstract** (accessed 07 April 2016).

CHAPTER 4 PRESCRIBING, CLINICAL PHARMACY AND ASEPTIC SERVICES VERIFICATION

Prescribing of aseptically-prepared medicines requires all the care and attention which would normally be accorded to any prescribing activity, and the nature of the products and routes of administration also bring additional risks. Risks exist from inadvertent administration by the incorrect route e.g. inappropriate intrathecal administration of vinca alkaloids (NPSA 2008), from inappropriate rate of infusion or dilution e.g. potassium (NPSA 2002) or neonatal parenteral nutrition (PN) (DH 2011), and the inherent toxicity of cytotoxic drugs. Checks of the prescription during the clinical pharmacy and aseptic services verification processes are required to reduce these risks and to ensure that the prepared medicines are appropriate for the patient. For the purposes of these standards these checks will be referred to as 'clinical pharmacy verification' and 'aseptic services verification'. It is recognised that there are other terms in common use to describe these processes e.g. 'clinical checking' or 'screening of prescriptions' or 'prescription validation' etc. The checks required and terminology used may vary according to the medicine, route and organisational arrangements.

4.1 Prescribing

4.1.1 All prescriptions should be signed by an approved prescriber who has successfully completed appropriate training. This may be a doctor or non-medical prescriber.

4.1.2 A current approved list of non-medical prescribers should be available.

4.1.3 Organisational policies and associated procedures should be available and adhered to cover the following where applicable:

- Prescribing preparation and administration of Injectable Medicines (NPSA 2007)
- Prescribing of paediatric and neonatal Parenteral Nutrition (DH 2011)
- Prescribing of adult Parenteral Nutrition
- Prescribing of Chemotherapy (DH 2014)
- Prescribing and use of Unlicensed Medicines (MHRA 2014)
- Prescribing of Radiopharmaceuticals (ARSAC 2014)
- Intrathecal chemotherapy (DH 2008 and local organisational policy)
- Intravenous Administration of Potassium (NPSA 2002).

These policies, that may be available separately or in combination in an overall medicines policy, should clearly define the roles and responsibilities of doctors, pharmacists and other healthcare professionals in the prescribing of aseptic products. A multi-disciplinary approach to prescribing of PN should be considered (see Chapter 3: Minimising risk with injectable medicines).

4.1.4 All staff involved in any stage of the prescribing and verification processes should have ready access to appropriate information and reference sources when undertaking these tasks. This should include the current *British National Formulary* and an injectable medicine guide (local guidelines or a database such as the *NHS Injectable Medicines Guide.* **www.medusa.wales.nhs.uk**). For clinical trials, a copy of the current approved protocol should be available.

4.1.5 Prescribing for paediatric and neonatal patients should be made with reference to specialised neonatal and paediatric dose guidelines. This should include the *BNF for Children* (current edition).

4.1.6 All chemotherapy regimens should be documented and authorised by the appropriate multidisciplinary team (MDT), or consultant or follow an approved trial protocol.

    4.1.6.1 This document should include details of:

- critical tests required
- cumulative doses for specific named drugs
- regimen and individual drug identification
- diluents and dilution volumes, and any hydrations
- supportive drugs
- administration route and duration.

    4.1.6.2 In the event of a deviation from the agreed algorithms there should be a procedure for recording this and it should include:

- the regimen used or change in order of the regimens
- the reason for the deviation.

    4.1.6.3 There should be a document control system to ensure the current approved versions of regimens are in use (see Chapter 8: Pharmaceutical Quality System) although this might not be under the control of the aseptic unit.

4.1.7 Radiopharmaceuticals are Prescription Only Medicines. Therapeutic radiopharmaceuticals and certain radioactive medical devices should be requested and approved on an individual patient basis by the Administration of Radioactive Substances Advisory Committee (ARSAC 2014) certificate holder for that therapy.

Requests received in nuclear medicine departments for diagnostic procedures are often for a named procedure rather than for a particular radiopharmaceutical and so may not include all on the information that would be required on a prescription.

4.1.7.1 Diagnostic radiopharmaceuticals may be supplied for use in specific patients against Nuclear Medicine requests provided that the following conditions are met:

- The request includes the patient details (as for a prescription)
- The request states which procedure is to be carried out
- The request has been approved for that procedure by an ARSAC certificate holder or their designated deputy, in compliance with *The Medicines (Administration of Radioactive Substances) Amendment Regulations 2006*
- A protocol is in place for the procedure which includes the name and dose of the radiopharmaceutical to be used
- The protocol has been approved by an ARSAC certificate holder and ratified by the organisation's Medicine Management Committee
- The requestor and/or the approver are named on the protocol and have been appropriately trained, with approval from the ARSAC certificate holder.

4.1.7.2 The pharmacist verifying the dose request should be familiar with the protocol for the procedure and confirm that the approver has authority to approve the request.

4.1.7.3 A number of nuclear medicine procedures require the administration of non-radioactive medicinal products in order to optimise the biodistribution of the radiopharmaceutical. The protocol for the procedure should clearly indicate the circumstances where these non-radioactive adjuncts can be prescribed.

4.1.8 All clinical trial protocols should be documented and authorised. There should be a document control system to ensure the current approved versions are in use (see Chapter 8: Pharmaceutical Quality System). The Accountable Pharmacist should ensure that the activities involved in the trial are in compliance with requirements of *The Medicines for Human Use (Clinical Trials) Regulations 2004*. In practice this means that no manufacture of an investigational medicinal product (IMP) as defined by *The Medicines for Human Use (Clinical Trials) Regulations 2004* can be carried out unless the site has a MIA(IMP) authorisation. Labelling may, however, be carried out without a MIA(IMP) authorisation if the requirements of the hospital exemption in Section 37 of this legislation are met.

4.1.9 Whether generated manually or electronically, prescriptions should be clear, unambiguous and accurate.

4.1.10 Approved standardised prescription formats should be used for each product type.

4.1.11 Where a computerised system is used for prescribing or dose calculations, the system and all of its outputs should be fully validated (see Part B – 2.6) before being put into routine use. In addition:

- The roles and responsibilities of staff using the system should be clearly defined so that the status of the prescription is understood at all stages of the prescribing, validation and verification process
- Electronic prescribing systems should be subject to the same standards of security and viewed as having the same legal status as a paper prescription
- It should be possible to demonstrate a full audit trail of changes made to the electronic prescription and any associated calculations or doses.

4.2 Clinical pharmacy and aseptic services verification

4.2.1 The pharmacist in the aseptic unit may not be the most appropriate person to verify the prescription from a clinical perspective. Clinical pharmacy verification is the process of verifying against the prescription that the product is clinically appropriate for the particular patient and aseptic services verification is the process of verifying that the clinical pharmacy verification of the prescription has been carried out, that the prescribed constituents are compatible and the formulation is stable, and that the product is the correct presentation for the intended route of administration.

A pharmacist in the clinical area with a greater knowledge of the patient or with specialised clinical expertise may be better placed to perform the clinical verification. The clinical and aseptic services verification may, in certain cases, be carried out by the same person.

4.2.2　A written organisational policy and supporting procedures should be available and in use which cover the arrangements and accountability for clinical and aseptic services verification. For example, the roles and responsibilities of the nutrition team should be defined, if applicable. The policy should include the course of action if changes are made to the prescription by the pharmacist during either clinical pharmacy or aseptic services verification.

4.3　Clinical pharmacy verification

The checks required to clinically verify a prescription may vary according to the product type and individual medicine.

4.3.1　There should be clinical pharmacy verification procedures which include checks for the following against the **original** prescription:

- Prescriber's details and full signature (may be electronic if an electronic prescribing system is in use)
- Prescriber is authorised to prescribe the medicine(s) (e.g. chemotherapy should only be prescribed by authorised prescribers, paediatric and neonatal parenteral nutrition should be initiated by a senior clinician)
- Intrathecal chemotherapy is only prescribed by authorised prescribers on the Intrathecal Register
- Patient details (e.g. full name, hospital number, consultant, ward, date of birth)
- Patient demographics (age, height and weight) where appropriate have been correctly recorded on the prescription
- Where body surface area (BSA) or creatinine clearance (CrCl) is used in the dose calculation it has been correctly calculated, taking into account recent patient parameters
- Correct dose calculation
- Doses are appropriate with respect to renal and hepatic function and any experienced toxicities
- Drug interactions (including with food) or conflicts with patient allergies
- Method of administration is appropriate
- Administration details (route, diluent, volume, rate, duration).

For electronic systems there is no need to manually check calculations e.g. doses, BSA, CrCl etc. on each occasion so long as the electronic system has been appropriately validated (see Part B – 2.6).

4.3.2 Additional checks are also required for the following:

For chemotherapy additional checks should include (BOPA 2013):

- Where there is access to either clinic notes, treatment plan or electronic record on first cycle, check the regimen is intended treatment and is appropriate for patient's diagnosis, medical history, performance status and chemotherapy history
- The timing of administration is appropriate i.e. the interval since last treatment
- Cumulative dose and maximum individual dose as appropriate
- Reason for and consistency of any dose adjustments, e.g. reduction(s) or escalations and ensure the reason is documented
- Laboratory values e.g. full blood counts, urea and electrolytes and liver function tests are within accepted limits, if appropriate (see below)
- Other essential tests have been undertaken, if appropriate
- Supportive care e.g. anti-emetics, steroids etc. is prescribed and it is appropriate for the patient and regimen.

4.3.3 In general, chemotherapy doses should not be released from the aseptic unit until these checks are complete. However, some services may allow dose checking of prescriptions in advance without access to laboratory values. This may not take into account the patient's blood counts or toxicities and hence policies should be in place clearly defining who is responsible for checking full blood count results and monitoring toxicities for chemotherapy prepared in advance before administration is authorised.

4.3.4 For parenteral nutrition additional checks (DH 2011) are also required for the following:

- For paediatric and neonatal parenteral nutrition the prescription has been initiated by a senior clinician
- Where an individualised parenteral nutrition (as opposed to a standard formulation) is prescribed, it is clinically appropriate
- The route of administration is appropriate for the glucose concentration of the parenteral nutrition.

4.3.5 Technical issues such as the stability of components, the osmolality (see Chapter 6: Formulation, stability and shelf life) may require a modification of the prescription in the pharmacy aseptic unit. In this instance, a pharmacist familiar with PN should carry out the final verification of the amended regimen, discuss any changes with the prescriber if necessary and ensure they are recorded on the prescription.

4.3.6 For radiopharmaceuticals, additional checks (IR (MER) 2000) are also required:

- The patient radioactive dose prescribed is in accordance with the Diagnostic Reference Level for that procedure (ARSAC 2014)
- Paediatric radioactive dose prescribing is in accordance with national guidelines (ARSAC 2014)
- For certain procedures, that the patient's concomitant medication has been withheld or administered for the appropriate period prior to the procedure being undertaken.

4.3.7 If the prescription is not available in the unit at the time of preparation (e.g. use of facsimiles, scanned documents, order forms) there should be a robust system for ensuring that the above checks have been made against the original prescription before the product is released.

4.4 Aseptic services verification

4.4.1 The Authorised Pharmacist should carry out the aseptic services verification process and as part of this ensure that a clinical verification has been completed in accordance with the specific organisational policy.

4.4.2 The aseptic services verification should include the following checks:

- The prescription has been clinically verified
- The prescribed constituents are compatible and the formulation is stable (see Chapter 6: Formulation, stability and shelf life)
- The product is the correct presentation for the intended route of administration.

4.4.3 A record should be made on the worksheet indicating who carried out the verification of each prescription.

QUALITY ASSURANCE OF ASEPTIC PREPARATION SERVICES:
STANDARDS HANDBOOK PART A

References

Administration of Radioactive Substances Advisory Committee (ARSAC) (2014). *Notes for guidance on the Clinical Administration of Radiopharmaceuticals and Use of Sealed Radioactive Sources.* London: Administration of Radioactive Substances Advisory Committee. March 2006 (Revised 2014).

British Oncology Pharmacy Association (BOPA) (2013). *Standards for Pharmacy Verification of Prescriptions for Cancer Medicines.* British Oncology Pharmacy Association. Available at: ***www.bopawebsite.org*** (accessed 15 April 2016).

Department of Health (DH) (2008). *Updated National Guidance on Safe Administration of Intrathecal Chemotherapy.* HSC 2008/001. London: Department of Health.

Department of Health (DH) (2011). *Improving practice and reducing risk in the provision of parenteral nutrition for neonates and children.* Report from the Paediatric Chief Pharmacists Group. London: Department of Health. Available at: ***www.rpharms.com*** (accessed 04 April 2016).

Department of Health (DH) (2014). *Manual for Cancer Standards: Chemotherapy Measures.* v2.0. NHS England Gateway No.16104. London: National Peer Review Programme – National Cancer Action Team.

Joint Formulary Committee. *British National Formulary.* Current edn. London: BMJ Group and Pharmaceutical Press.

Medicines and Healthcare products Regulatory Agency (MHRA) (2014). *The supply of unlicensed medicinal product ("specials"). MHRA Guidance Note 14.* London: Medicines and Healthcare products Regulatory Agency. Available at: ***https://www.gov.uk/government/publications/supply-unlicensed-medicinal-products-specials*** (accessed 15 April 2016).

National Patient Safety Agency (2002). *Patient Safety Alert. Potassium chloride concentrate solutions.* London: National Patient Safety Agency.

National Patient Safety Agency (2007). *Patient Safety Alert. Promoting safer use of injectable medicines.* NPSA/2007/20. London: National Patient Safety Agency.

National Patient Safety Agency (NPSA) (2008). *Rapid Response Report. Using Vinca Alkaloid Minibags (Adult/ Adolescent Units)* NPSA/2008/RRR004. Available at: ***www.nrls.npsa.nhs.uk/alerts/?entryid45=59890&p=2*** (accessed 26 February 2016).

NHS Injectable Medicines Guide (Medusa) [online]. Available at: ***http://medusa.wales.nhs.uk*** (accessed 05 April 2016).

Paediatric Formulary Committee. *BNF for Children.* Current edn. London: BMJ Group, Pharmaceutical Press and RCPCH Publications.

The Ionising Radiations Regulations 1999. SI 1999 No.3232. London: The Stationery Office.

The Ionising Radiation (Medical Exposure) Regulations (IR(ME)R) 2000. SI 2000 No. 1059. London: The Stationery Office.

The Medicines (Administration of Radioactive Substances) Regulations 1978. SI 1978 No. 1006. London: HMSO.

The Medicines (Administration of Radioactive Substances) Amendment Regulations 2006. SI 2006 No. 2806. Available at: ***www.legislation.gov.uk/uksi/2006/2806/pdfs/uksi_20062806_en.pdf*** (accessed 13 April 2016).

The Medicines for Human Use (Clinical Trials) Regulations 2004. SI 2004 No.1031. London: The Stationery Office.

CHAPTER 5 MANAGEMENT

Aseptic units should ensure that the products they prepare are fit for their intended use, comply with the standards in this text, and do not place patients at risk due to inadequate safety or quality.

Achieving this objective is the responsibility of senior management and requires the commitment, understanding and participation of all staff who are involved in the ordering, preparation, storage and supply of aseptic products.

There should be a comprehensive and correctly implemented Pharmaceutical Quality System (PQS), incorporating the principles of Good Manufacturing Practice (GMP) (EC 2015) and quality risk management (EMA 2006).

The standards in this chapter are interrelated with those in Chapters 3, 8 and 9 on Minimising risk with injectable medicines, Pharmaceutical Quality System, and Personnel, training and competency assessment respectively.

5.1 General issues

5.1.1 All departments undertaking aseptic preparation activities should have an appropriate documented organisational structure that indicates clearly the responsibilities and accountability of each member of staff.

5.1.2 Aseptic units should be under the management of an Accountable Pharmacist who should ensure that a system of quality assurance is implemented that incorporates the principles set down in these standards. Routine monitoring of the adherence to procedures in the form of internal audit should be undertaken.

5.1.3 All staff working in the aseptic unit should be professionally accountable, either directly or indirectly, to the Accountable Pharmacist.

5.1.4 To assist Chief Pharmacists to discharge their overall responsibility for the PQS and associated quality indicator monitoring, the Accountable Pharmacist should be directly accountable to the Chief Pharmacist.

5.1.5 There should be a system for capturing staff suggestions for improvement and implementing regulatory changes.

5.1.6 All aseptic preparation should be carried out by, or under the supervision of, a pharmacist authorised by the Accountable Pharmacist. (The Accountable Pharmacist is also an Authorised Pharmacist by definition). Pharmacists supervising any aseptic preparation carried out outside normal working hours to the same quality system should be Authorised Pharmacists.

5.1.7 The responsibility for the release of an aseptically-prepared product should be taken by an accredited product approver in accordance with the criteria set down in Chapter 14: Product approval. This may not necessarily be the same Authorised Pharmacist who supervised the preparation of the product.

5.1.8 The Accountable Pharmacist should authorise the Standard Operating Procedures. Any deviation from these procedures should be approved and should be fully documented in accordance with the PQS.

5.1.9 Senior managers should ensure that all staff who are involved in the preparation and supply of aseptically-prepared products clearly understand their level of responsibility and accountability, and are competent to carry out their role.

5.1.10 The Chief Pharmacist has overall responsibility for medicines management within the organisation. In practice, this means that they are ultimately responsible for ensuring that effective governance arrangements are in place across the organisation for all injectable medicines, whether prepared in clinical areas, in pharmacy or outsourced.

5.1.11 The Chief Pharmacist holds ultimate responsibility for the adequate resourcing of the aseptic preparation service to ensure that it meets the defined national standards as described in this text. This needs to be formally documented in an organisational policy (such as the injectable medicines policy).

5.1.12 The Chief Pharmacist is also responsible for ensuring that a policy on aseptic preparation is in place and that, where this allows delegated product approval in line with Nationally Recognised Competency Framework requirements (ASAWG 2014), this has specific, formal, organisation board-level agreement.

5.1.13 There should be an appropriate reporting structure so that all accredited product approvers are accountable directly to the Accountable Pharmacist for this activity and that this is reflected in their job description (see Chapter 14: Product approval).

5.1.14 Where delegated product approval is in place, the Chief Pharmacist and Accountable Pharmacist should agree a suitable management structure within the aseptic unit to ensure that the requirements of the Nationally Recognised Competency Framework (ASAWG 2014) are met at all times that the unit is operational.

5.2 Pharmaceutical Quality System

5.2.1 The PQS (see Chapter 8: Pharmaceutical Quality System) should be fully documented and its effectiveness monitored.

5.2.2 All elements of the PQS should be adequately resourced with competent personnel, suitable and sufficient equipment and facilities.

5.2.3 Senior managers should ensure that quality indicators, e.g. complaints, errors, microbiological non-conformances, are recorded, investigated and regularly trended. Any adverse trends should be acted on in a timely manner.

5.2.4 There should be regular (normally monthly) quality management meetings to review the PQS. It is the responsibility of the Chief Pharmacist to ensure that there are adequate resources to enable this review to take place. The Chief Pharmacist should be aware whether the quality system is functioning correctly, e.g. by participation in, or reports from, these meetings. An example agenda would include: deviations; change controls; errors; complaints; capacity; audit (internal and external); microbiological out-of-specifications; planned preventative maintenance (PPM) for facilities and equipment.

5.2.5 Units should continually review their PQS to ensure that standards of quality are maintained. Should circumstances arise where this is no longer the case, the Chief Pharmacist should take a risk management approach, which may include implementing contingency plans, to ensure that patient safety and continuity of care are not compromised (see Chapter 3: Minimising risk with injectable medicines).

5.2.6 There should be a culture of continuous, quality improvement in the department. Sharing best practice and learning from errors (both internal and external to the department) to optimise patient care associated with aseptically-prepared medicines should be accepted practice.

5.2.7 The Accountable Pharmacist should authorise documented procedures for product preparation and these procedures should be readily available. These procedures should be based on evaluated data but if no data are available the decision to prepare the product should be made in the context of the clinical needs of the patient and the potential risks.

5.2.8 If a product is requested outside the PQS, i.e. a non-catalogue request, it is the responsibility of the Authorised Pharmacist to consider the risk/benefit for the patient in the context of their clinical needs. Appropriate risk management arrangement should be in place.

5.2.9 If, under exceptional circumstances, an Authorised Pharmacist decides, using the criteria in Chapter 3, to prepare a product for which there are no documented procedures, he/she should take full responsibility for the quality of that product and the procedures used for preparation should be fully documented, along with the rationale for preparation. The Authorised Pharmacist should inform the Accountable Pharmacist of this at the earliest opportunity.

5.3 Audit

5.3.1 It is the responsibility of the Chief Pharmacist to ensure that internal audits of aseptic preparation are carried out on a regular basis. Any faults or deficiencies, however identified, should be promptly rectified. (See Chapter 16: Internal and external audit.)

5.3.2 It is the joint responsibility of the Chief Pharmacist and the Regional Quality Assurance Specialists to ensure that external audits are carried out in accordance with current NHS requirements (NHS Executive 1997).

5.3.3 The Chief Pharmacist is responsible for ensuring that an action plan to address the deficiencies is sent to the external auditor in a timely manner and that actions are completed within the agreed timescale. The Chief Pharmacist is also responsible for communicating to the external auditor any major changes to facilities, key personnel etc., or slippage of the action plan.

5.3.4 It is the responsibility of the Chief Pharmacist to ensure that quality assurance systems are regularly reviewed and that any off-site testing is regularly audited.

5.3.5 The Chief Pharmacist is responsible for regulatory compliance. For example, in accordance with *The Medicines for Human Use (Clinical Trials) Regulations 2004*, manufacture of an investigation medicinal product requires an MIA (IMP) (see Part B – 6).

5.4 Contingency planning

5.4.1 There should be a detailed contingency plan to cover any unforeseen event, e.g. unavailability of key personnel etc. that could lead to shutdown of the unit, or temporary unavailability of the service. The contingency plan should include the details of who to contact in the event of failure. The contingency plan should include business continuity, e.g. the use of alternative aseptic facilities, outsourcing etc. Risk reduction measures, such as review of shelf life and storage conditions, may be necessary.

5.5 Capacity planning

5.5.1 The Chief Pharmacist should ensure that the department has a current and effectively implemented capacity plan (see Part B – 5).

5.5.2 The Chief Pharmacist is responsible for ensuring that the capacity plan is approved by senior hospital management external to pharmacy, for example at board level, to enable it to be effective at managing pharmacy workload in the context of the organisation's injectable medicines policy.

5.5.3 Workload figures should be regularly reviewed (suggested monthly) against this plan and action taken where appropriate. Significant variations should be authorised by senior managers within the organisation, under change control.

5.5.4 The capacity plan should have the following attributes:

- It should ensure adequate resourcing for the expected demand.
- There should be a thorough understanding of demand and preparation constraints, and appropriate strategies to highlight imbalances in a timely manner to effect appropriate action.
- It should address the entire scope of work undertaken in the aseptic unit, including essential underpinning tasks such as maintenance of the PQS.
- If aseptic services staff are involved with dispensing outsourced aseptic products, this should be included in the capacity plan.

5.5.5 The capacity plan should be reviewed at least annually or when there are significant changes to supply and demand. Any changes should be managed via the change control system.

References

European Commission (2015). *The rules governing medicinal products in the European Community. Vol IV. Good Manufacturing Practice for medicinal products.* Available at: ***http://ec.europa.eu/health/documents/eudralex/vol-4/index_en.htm*** (accessed 26 February 2016).

European Medicines Agency (EMA) (2006). *International Committee on Harmonisation (ICH) Guideline Q9 on Quality Risk Management.* EMA/CHMP/ICH/24235/2006. London: European Medicines Agency.

NHS Aseptic Services Accreditations Working Group (ASAWG) (2014). *Nationally Recognised Competency Framework for Pharmacists and Pharmacy Technicians: Product Approval (Release) in Aseptic Services under Section 10 Exemption.* Available at: ***www.nhspedc.nhs.uk/supports.htm*** (accessed 25 February 2016).

NHS Executive (1997). *Executive Letter (97) 52: Aseptic Dispensing in NHS Hospitals.* London: Department of Health.

The Medicines for Human Use (Clinical Trials) Regulations 2004. SI 2004 No.1031. London: The Stationery Office.

CHAPTER 6 FORMULATION, STABILITY AND SHELF LIFE

Expiry periods (shelf lives) given to products should be evaluated in accordance with the local conditions and formulations. Data obtained from the literature or from the starting material manufacturer should be carefully assessed to ensure their appropriateness to the local situation.

Under no circumstances should an expiry period of seven days be exceeded for products prepared in unlicensed aseptic units (see Chapter 3: Minimising risk with injectable medicines). As a general principle, the shortest expiry period consistent with the intended usage pattern of the product should be used. Use of the shortest possible shelf life does not obviate the need to comply fully with the standards described in this text.

The overall aim should be to minimise the time between preparation of the product and its administration so that the opportunity for any live microorganisms inadvertently introduced into the product to multiply is restricted and levels of degradation are also minimised.

The range of formulations encountered during aseptic preparation is broad and ranges from fairly simple two-constituent systems to complex mixtures with in excess of 50 starting materials, e.g. parenteral nutrition (PN) regimens, and from simple, well-understood small molecules to complex biopharmaceuticals.

Product shelf life should be assigned to ensure the quality of the product is suitable for the patient at the time of administration. The assignment of a shelf life can be a complex process even for small molecules and is extremely complex for parenteral nutrition and for biopharmaceuticals.

6.1   Stability testing

6.1.1   Where stability studies are to be carried out in-house or specifically commissioned then the standards outlined in *A Standard Protocol for Deriving and Assessment of Stability Part 1 – Aseptic Preparations (small molecules)* (PQAC 2015a), *Part 2 – Aseptic Preparations (Biopharmaceuticals)* (PQAC 2015b), or *Part 4 – Parenteral Nutrition* (PQAC 2016) should be followed.

6.1.2   It should be borne in mind that even if a full in-house stability study is not possible, ongoing information in support of a shelf life assigned can be obtained by testing products at the end of their shelf life by stability-indicating methods. This should be used to provide additional information to published studies or, in extreme circumstances, to provide assurance of an extrapolation that has been carried out.

6.2 Sources of information

6.2.1 Many sources of stability information exist, some more reliable than others. It is the responsibility of the Authorised Pharmacist to ensure that the information used is scientifically valid and relevant to the local circumstances. Further guidance is given below.

6.2.2 A number of texts are available through quality control and medicines information, including textbooks, product data sheets and published research papers. The manufacturer's SmPC is a prime source of information as this has been reviewed as part of the product licensing process. Often, however, the data is quite limited and aseptic units may need to rely on published or peer-reviewed studies for extended data. General reference sources, such as textbooks, should be used with care and the applicability of the data to the actual brands of products used should be carefully assessed.

6.2.3 For PN, the prime source of information should be the supplier of the major starting materials (amino acid and lipid solutions). A matrix approach should be taken with PN, where all starting materials need to be within pre-defined limits in order to assure stability. It would generally be expected to use the major starting materials, such as amino acids and lipids, from the same manufacturer.

6.2.4 Where a computerised system is used to perform stability calculations (for example, while compounding PN) appropriate validation (see Part B – 2.6) commensurate with the level of risk should be performed on the system, ideally using known stability problems to ensure that the output of the calculations is correct. The use of a computerised system should supplement, and not replace, the professional judgement of a member of staff skilled in formulation and stability assessment.

6.2.5 Suitable data should be sought and evaluated before products are prepared. This data should be retained on file, together with the record of its assessment.

6.2.6 If no data is available, the decision to prepare should be made in the context of the clinical needs of the patient and this risk assessment should be fully documented. This should only occur in exceptional circumstances.

6.2.7 If a product made under the circumstances described above is to continue being prepared in the aseptic unit, then appropriate stability data should be obtained or generated to support the shelf life assigned.

6.3 Data interpretation

6.3.1 Data from information sources needs to be interpreted for the local situation; in general data should only be used for the specific brands, concentrations, diluents and containers that are quoted in the reference. Studies should be checked for compliance with standards (PQAC 2015a and PQAC 2015b).

6.3.2 Generally data can be safely interpolated, for example to any concentrations between the low and high concentrations which have given suitable stability profiles, however care should be taken with biopharmaceuticals (see below).

6.3.3 Extrapolation should only be done where there is a good understanding of the product stability and degradation profile and, for example, the characteristics of various container systems that may be required. Stability of biopharmaceuticals can be influenced by how they are handled and other factors such as the final container, the amount of air present in the final container and the amount of silicone oil in syringes. There should therefore be no extrapolation of data for biopharmaceuticals.

6.3.4 For biopharmaceuticals, units using published or peer-reviewed studies to support an expiry period beyond that stated in the SmPC should ensure that they are using identical practices to those in the study for preparation, storage and transportation with identical starting materials, consumables and storage containers.

6.3.5 The levels, nature and potential toxicity of any degradation products should be considered as part of shelf life assessment.

6.4 Factors affecting stability

Factors which may have an impact on product stability are discussed further below.

6.4.1 Chemical degradation
The main mechanisms of chemical degradation for small molecules are hydrolysis, oxidation and photolysis. Other degradation pathways, e.g. polymerisation and isomerisation, can also occur. For biopharmaceuticals, the situation is highly complex and can include chemical changes, conformational changes, aggregation, fragmentation and interactions with containers and excipients.

6.4.2 Concentration of active components

Concentration can either enhance or reduce stability. For example, Ampicillin degrades more quickly in high concentrations. Oxidation and photodegradation reactions generally follow zero order kinetics and so medicines degraded in this way often have a shorter shelf life at lower concentrations.

6.4.3 pH

The rates of degradation of many drugs are pH dependent. Buffering, or the lack of buffering ability, may have a significant impact on stability.

6.4.4 Diluent / vehicle

Some drugs can be diluted in various diluents but stability is often significantly different in each, for example Cisplatin needs the presence of chloride ions to remain stable.

6.4.5 Catalysis

Some ingredients in formulations can act as catalysts for the breakdown of other ingredients. For example copper ions from trace metal additions in PN preparations catalyse the oxidation of Ascorbic Acid; buffer ions may catalyse the hydrolysis of penicillins.

6.4.6 Ionic strength

The reaction rate may be influenced by the ionic strength of the medium, but this is usually a less important factor than the other factors given above.

6.4.7 Preparation process

The method of preparation can be critical to stability. The correct order of mixing of materials in PN compounding is essential to avoid high concentrations of electrolytes, which affect lipid particle size, and also to avoid high concentrations of divalent metal ions mixing with phosphate, which could cause precipitation.

Biopharmaceuticals are susceptible to changes in handling, which include the level of shaking, contact with components, needle sizes, filtering etc.

6.4.8 Photosensitivity

There can be significant photodegradation of some drugs, e.g. Carmustine. It is important that this is understood and the impact of any light protective wraps is also assessed.

6.4.9 Filters

Filters used in preparation processes can cause problems such as adsorption onto the filter medium that will reduce the potency of some injections. Hence, care should be taken to assess the impact of the use of filters in preparation and also in administration.

6.4.10 Containers

The nature of the container can contribute to stability of the product in a number of ways including:

- by releasing leachable chemicals (e.g. plasticisers and lubricants from rubber stoppers)
- by interacting with the product, for example lubricants may interact with monoclonal antibodies
- by sorption of ingredients from the solution into or onto the container.

There may also be differences in container permeability, allowing gaseous diffusion into the container (important for products which are susceptible to oxidation) and increased water loss leading to concentration of solutions.

6.5 Storage

In accordance with advice in other parts of this handbook (see Chapter 15: Storage and distribution), products should be stored in a refrigerator where this does not impact on quality. In general, low storage temperatures slow down chemical degradation, sorption, etc. However, it should be remembered that low-temperature storage can result in physical instability, e.g. precipitation, such as in Aciclovir infusions. The converse can also be true though: phosphates are less soluble at room or body temperature, which has led to precipitation in PN solution once it is removed from the refrigerator.

6.6 Microbiological and container integrity issues

6.6.1 Aseptic preparation facilities should enable the preparation of injections in controlled environments with a high level of sterility assurance. The integrity of the final container should have been assessed up to the shelf life that individual products are assigned. For single component systems, such as infusion bags, this can take the form of a check for leaks but for multiple component systems, such as capped syringes, there needs to be an assessment of container integrity.

6.6.2 Ideally, this should take the form of in-house integrity testing in accordance with *Protocols for the Integrity Testing of Syringes* (PQAC 2013).

As a minimum, nationally collated data should be reviewed and its applicability to the specific syringe/closure combinations/fill volumes in use should be assessed alongside in-house broth transfer test data.

6.6.3 In order to maintain microbiological integrity, infusion bags should not be spiked ahead of the time of their use in clinical areas.

6.7 Expiry period

6.7.1 The expiry period of the product should be based on all of the information available. Specific pieces of information should not be ignored and should form part of the assessment; this includes physico-chemical stability and microbiological contamination risks.

6.7.2 For biopharmaceuticals, it is particularly important that other investigators' findings are considered alongside any in-house data, specifically where these findings may ask questions of the validity of the data from the in-house study.

6.7.3 The expiry period should be reviewed and reassessed if new data becomes available relevant to the product.

6.7.4 The expiry period should not exceed seven days in any circumstances in an unlicensed aseptic unit.

6.8 Control of procurement contract changes for starting materials and components

Changes to starting materials and key components should be fully assessed using a formal change control procedure before they are introduced (see Chapter 8: Pharmaceutical Quality System). Stability information is often specific to a particular manufacturer of starting material and, hence, a new shelf life assessment will be required when this changes; this re-assessment should be recorded. The document *Assessment of shelf life following a change in supplier of starting material* (R and D 2012) provides further guidance and examples.

6.9 Stability file

6.9.1 Stability data, including copies of studies used and in-house assessments, should be maintained by a controlled system in a stability file (paper-based or electronic folder) for ease of reference.

6.9.2 Worksheets should have stability references which cross-reference to the data and assessments held in the stability file.

6.10 Pharmacovigilance

Any problems with products or patient adverse drug reactions should be investigated thoroughly. This investigation should lead to a review of the assigned formulation, storage conditions and shelf life where appropriate. Reporting of such issues should be encouraged within the organisation, for example via the Datix system.

References

NHS National Pharmaceutical Research and Development Group (R and D) (2012). *Aseptic medicinal products; Assessment of shelf life following a change in supplier of starting material.* Proceedings of the NHS National Pharmaceutical Research and Development Group.

NHS Pharmaceutical Quality Assurance Committee (PQAC) (2013). *Protocols for the Integrity Testing of Syringes.* 2nd edn. Microbiology Protocols Group and NHS Pharmaceutical Research and Development Group (R and D).

NHS Pharmaceutical Quality Assurance Committee (PQAC) (2015a). *A Standard Protocol for Deriving and Assessment of Stability Part 1 - Aseptic Preparations (small molecules).* 3rd edn. NHS National Pharmaceutical Research and Development Group.

NHS Pharmaceutical Quality Assurance Committee (PQAC) (2015b). *A Standard Protocol for Deriving and Assessment of Stability Part 2 - Aseptic Preparations (Biopharmaceuticals).* 2nd edn. NHS National Pharmaceutical Research and Development Group.

NHS Pharmaceutical Quality Assurance Committee (PQAC) (2016). *A Standard Protocol for Derivation and Assessment of Stability Part 4 – Parenteral Nutrition.* NHS National Research and Development Group.

CHAPTER 7 FACILITIES AND EQUIPMENT

Facilities and equipment should be located, designed, constructed, adapted and maintained to suit the operations to be carried out. Their layout and/or design should aim to minimise the risk of errors and permit effective cleaning and maintenance in order to avoid cross-contamination, build-up of dust or dirt and, in general, any adverse effect on the quality of products (EC 2015).

7.1 Design principles for new or refurbished facilities and equipment

7.1.1 The performance criteria of the new facility or new item of critical equipment (such as, isolators, refrigerators etc.) should be established prior to building or installation by the development of a detailed user requirements specification (URS). The URS should be part of an overarching change control for the project that takes into account knowledge of deviations, errors and malfunctions of the previous existing facilities and processes (EC 2015 Annex 15).

7.1.2 Compliance to this previously defined design specification or URS should be confirmed through a series of validation stages which will include design, installation, operational and performance qualification, (DQ, IQ, OQ, PQ), supporting subsequent process validation (PV). The qualification protocols should be approved by the Accountable Pharmacist, including those drawn up by any external contractor providing validation services.

Current standards need to be knowledgeably interpreted, and future developments considered before the URS is finalised. Of particular importance is due consideration of current and future capacity and workforce requirements. Sufficient resources (time, funding, personnel and expertise) should be allocated for validation activities (Beaney 2010).

7.1.3 The approach to validation should be detailed as part of the comprehensive Validation Master Plan (VMP). This should also be subject to the deviation and change control systems. (See Chapter 8: Pharmaceutical Quality System).

7.1.4 Each stage of the validation process should be defined in a validation protocol which should be approved and authorised by the appropriate personnel as defined in the VMP. The continued maintenance of the facility or equipment should be considered as part of the VMP (EC 2015 Annex 15).

(Qualifications documents may be combined in some cases e.g. IQ and OQ for small projects.)

7.1.5 It should be clear at which point final handover into use is accepted and this should be documented and signed by the contractor performing the qualification and the personnel defined in the VMP, including the Accountable Pharmacist.

7.1.6 Any planned changes to the facilities, equipment or utilities which may affect the quality of the product should be formally assessed via the change control system.

7.1.7 Facilities and equipment should be designed to allow preparation to take place in areas connected in a logical order. Consideration needs to be given to the workflow of materials, finished products, personnel and waste.

7.1.8 Health and safety should also be considered in the design of a new facility, for example the provision of adequate extraction for disinfectants.

7.1.9 All clean rooms and clean air devices should be independently qualified by the purchaser or by a contractor acting on their behalf. They should subsequently be monitored at regular intervals (see Chapter 11: Monitoring).

7.1.10 All aseptic operations should be performed in a critical zone environment conforming to EU GMP Grade A (EC 2015). This should be located in a clean room, conforming to the correct standard, as defined in section 7.3. All classified rooms in the aseptic suite should conform to EU GMP (EC 2015, BSI 1999).

The critical zone environment may be provided by a clean air device such as:

- a unidirectional air flow workstation (UDAF)
- a pharmaceutical isolator.

There are various design types that will provide these conditions, e.g. horizontal or vertical laminar air flow cabinets, Class II safety cabinets, cytotoxic cabinets, negative and positive pressure isolators.

A well designed and maintained air handling unit (AHU/HVAC) is fundamental to the satisfactory operation of the facility and the AHU should comply with current NHS standards (DH 2007).

7.1.11 All areas used for preparation and storage should allow the orderly and logical positioning of equipment and materials.

Adequate segregation is required to minimise the risk of confusion between different products or components in order to avoid cross contamination and mix-up.

7.1.12 The facility walls, floors and ceilings of the classified environment should be smooth, impervious to fluids, resistant to sanitisation agents, and free from cracks and open joints. There should be an absence of exposed wood throughout the unit. Surfaces should not shed particulate matter and should permit easy, effective sanitisation. The joints between ceilings, walls and floor should be coved (EC 2015, BSI 1999).

7.1.13 Vision panels, switches, lights, intercoms, etc. should be flush fitting and easily cleanable. (The use of stainless steel is more expensive but more durable.)

Electrical trunking should be flush where possible, or at least have a sloping upper surface that aids easy cleaning and prevents accumulation of dust.

The replacement of light fittings (e.g. light bulbs and tubes) should be achievable without breaching the integrity of the clean room suite.

7.1.14 Clean rooms and support rooms should have a filtered air supply that maintains a positive pressure and air flow relative to surrounding areas of a lower grade and should flush the area effectively. In routine use, classified adjacent rooms should achieve a minimum differential pressure of 10 Pascals, and a minimum of 15 Pascals to an unclassified area (see Chapter 11: Monitoring).

It is advised that the design specification is at least 50% more than the minimum pressure differential.

7.1.15 Pressure differential readings between clean rooms and support rooms and from the clean room facility to external areas should be constantly indicated.

7.1.16 Pressure differentials should be constantly indicated across at least one typical HEPA filter supplying the clean rooms.

7.1.17 Air flow patterns should not create any dead spots or standing vortices. Determination of air flow patterns should be carried out on commissioning and after any significant modification to the room or cabinet. For EU Grade B (EC 2015) rooms and all types of clean air device, air flow pattern tests should be carried out annually as part of recommissioning (see Chapter 11: Monitoring).

7.1.18 The AHU should be designed to provide continuous compliance with the requirement for a minimum of 20 air changes per hour in all EU GMP Grade C and D (EC 2015) rooms and 30 air changes per hour in EU GMP Grade B (EC 2015) rooms (see Chapter 11: Monitoring).

This will typically allow the short clean-up period of less than 15 to 20 minutes (EC 2015).

7.1.19 There should be visible and audible alarms to indicate malfunction or failure of the air handling plant. The indicator board should be located at the entrance to the facility to ensure staff are aware of plant failure before entering (Beaney 2010).

The alarm system should also indicate malfunction or failure of the aseptic suite that occurred out of normal working hours and should require manual resetting.

7.1.20 Dispersed oil particulate (DOP) challenge access points should be carefully considered at the design stage. The injection points should be sufficient distance upstream from the terminal HEPA filters to allow uniform challenge (at least 15 duct widths from the filters) and should be located outside the clean areas. Upstream DOP concentration test points should also be provided.

7.1.21 Sinks and hand wash-stations should not be present in the clean room suite, except in exceptional circumstances. A formal hand wash prior to entry to the clean room suite is required. It is desirable to locate the hand wash facility adjacent to the entrance to the clean room suite.

7.1.22 Where it is considered necessary, after risk assessment, to site a sink within the aseptic facility e.g. radiopharmacy units, the location and use of the sink should be carefully considered in view of the potential to cause microbiological contamination. Regular monitoring and disinfection of the sink should be carried out (see Chapter 11: Monitoring).

7.1.23 Wall-mounted dispensers should be avoided in change rooms as they could result in damage to walls if changed and/or difficulty in cleaning.

7.2 General considerations

7.2.1 Clean rooms and clean air devices should run continuously, except during certain cleaning and maintenance activities. Requalification may be required after the activity. Aseptic manipulation should not be carried out until a satisfactory environment has been re-established, as verified by appropriate validation studies.

It is not desirable to operate a clean room with variable air change rates (in particular, operational setback as an energy saving measure is not acceptable) because it is necessary to maintain the operational status of the clean rooms to prevent accidental ingress of external contamination. If variable conditions are to be considered, these should ensure that the minimum operational standards are maintained; i.e. room overpressures remain above minimum standards and cleanup rates are similarly preserved. This should be subject to continuous monitoring (see Chapter 11: Monitoring).

7.2.2   All clean rooms and clean air devices should be cleaned regularly and frequently in accordance with an agreed written procedure. The procedure should require written confirmation that cleaning has been carried out and which cleaning agent was used (see Chapter 12: Cleaning, sanitisation and biodecontamination).

7.2.3   Critical equipment, including air-handling systems, isolators, cabinets, filling pumps, automated compounding systems, radiopharmaceutical calibrators, QC equipment etc. should be operated in accordance with SOPs and should be subject to commissioning and have a documented, planned preventative maintenance (PPM) and calibration schedule.

7.2.4   When monitoring indicates a loss of environmental control, or trend towards this, an impact assessment, root cause analysis and corrective and/ or preventative actions (CAPA) should be undertaken (see Chapter 8: Pharmaceutical Quality System).

7.2.5   The operational characteristics (the normal operating parameters) of the facilities and equipment should be confirmed following any planned or unplanned maintenance, i.e. the systems match the parameters established during initial validation.

7.2.6   Reports from service and maintenance visits should be reviewed and accepted by the Accountable Pharmacist in a timely manner, ideally upon receipt, to ensure that the correct level of testing has been applied in accordance with the relevant standards and that the unit complies with these standards. Checks should be documented.

7.2.7   Access to the facility and plant rooms housing the AHU/HVAC systems should be controlled and restricted to authorised personnel. A permit to work system should be in place and strictly enforced. Maintenance or recalibration of systems or equipment should not be undertaken without the documented approval of the Accountable Pharmacist.

7.2.8 The permit to work should detail all work to be undertaken and should be signed again by a senior member of the aseptic team on completion of the work. There should be formal acceptance back into operation after any necessary cleaning of the facility has been undertaken (see Chapter 12: Cleaning, sanitisation and biodecontamination).

7.3   Clean rooms and support rooms

The support room should be appropriately designed and provide adequate space. It is essential that the flow of work, personnel and waste is designed to minimise error, unnecessary crossover and to make efficient use of the space.

Siting equipment in rooms of the appropriate classification

Clean rooms housing clean air devices should be dedicated to aseptic preparation and all other activity should be forbidden.

7.3.1 Unidirectional air flow workstations (cabinets) should be located in a room classified to EU GMP Grade B (EC 2015) and accessed via an appropriate 3-stage change process. The air flow should be considered carefully and workstations positioned to ensure that contra flows do not occur.

7.3.2 Pharmaceutical isolators should be located in a room classified to a minimum of EU GMP Grade D (EC 2015) and accessed via an appropriate 2-stage change process.

7.3.3 Clean rooms should be entered through a changing room, the doors to which should be interlocked. The change room should be flushed effectively with directly filtered air supplied by a ceiling mounted HEPA filter on the clean side of the room.

7.3.4 The changing rooms should be divided by a suitable barrier, or equivalent, separating the space into a clean side and a 'dirty' side.

7.3.5 The final stage of the change area should, in the 'at rest' state, be the same grade as the area into which it leads (EC 2015).

7.3.6 Goods and materials should enter via a separate route to personnel.

7.3.7 The EU GMP Grade B (EC 2015) clean room should have an associated support room classified to a minimum of EU GMP Grade D (EC 2015) which is accessed via an appropriate 2-stage change process.

This area may be used for the storage and assembly of starting materials and components ready for transfer into the clean room.

7.3.8 The EU GMP Grade D (EC 2015) clean room should have an associated support room.

The support room should maintain a minimum of EU GMP Grade D (EC 2015) at rest.

This area may be used for the short-term storage and assembly of starting materials and components ready for transfer into the clean room.

7.3.9 Materials transferred into the support room should be subjected to a decarding and sanitisation process (see Chapter 12: Cleaning, sanitisation and biodecontamination). Transfer of materials should be through a dedicated hatch or hatches.

7.3.10 Ideally there should be dedicated in and out hatches. Alternatively segregation of products in and out can be managed by physical separation such as shelves.

7.3.11 All hatches should be fitted with interlocking doors and flushed with air flow sufficient to enable drying of disinfectants and the removal of particles (see Chapter 12: Cleaning, sanitisation and biodecontamination).

7.4 Clean rooms for specialist applications

7.4.1 Additional considerations should be taken into account for some clean rooms, including those used to prepare Advanced Therapy Medicinal Products (ATMPs). For example, gene therapy medicines require preparation in facilities designed to provide physical, chemical and biological barriers or any combination of these to limit contact with, and to provide a high level of protection for, personnel and the environment, depending on their classification. The most appropriate facilities and their location should be determined by risk assessment. (See Part B – 6, EC 2015 Annex 2).

7.4.2 Consideration should be given, in the risk assessment, to the necessity for a dedicated negative pressure isolator in a minimum EU GMP Grade D (EC 2015) background or Class II safety cabinet in a EU GMP Grade B (EC 2015) background. Dedicated equipment may be required depending on the specific nature of the materials being handled.

7.4.3 In certain circumstances it may be permissible for products of this nature, and other products intended for short term use, (shelf life restricted to 24 hours) to be prepared in isolators located in background environments that do not meet the required standard indicated in Part B – 6.

This should only be in response to an exceptional circumstance, and never routine practice. This should be accompanied by a formal, documented risk assessment (see Part B – 4).

7.4.4   There should be separate facilities for blood labelling in radiopharmacy (MHRA 2015, DH 2013, UKRG 2009).

   7.4.4.1   Facilities designed for radiopharmaceutical preparations should comply with the standards contained within *Quality Assurance of Radiopharmaceuticals* (UKRG 2012).

7.4.5   Facilities for PET/Cyclotrons require specialist expertise. More information is available in *Sampson's Textbook of Radiopharmacy* (Theobald 2011) and from the Institute of Physics and Engineering (IPEM) and the European Association of Nuclear Medicine (EANM).

7.5   Quality control facilities

7.5.1   Facilities used for processing samples should be physically separated from aseptic preparation but under the managerial control of the Chief Pharmacist or Quality Controller, or through a contract laboratory via a service and technical agreement (see Part B – 3 and Chapter 5: Management).

7.6   Equipment

The type of clean air device chosen should take into account the nature of the materials to be handled, considering both product and operator protection.

7.6.1   **Unidirectional air flow cabinets**
   As indicated in 7.3.1 above, the position of the cabinet within the room is crucial to the cabinet's correct function. Consideration should be given to the air flow within the clean room to minimise any interference in cabinet air flow, such as can be found if located too close to a door, for example.

   7.6.1.1   Air flows within the cabinets and clean room should not create any dead spots or standing vortices. The air flow patterns should be determined on commissioning and after any significant modifications. (See 7.1.17).

   7.6.1.2   All materials and components required for preparation should be transferred into the cabinet, in accordance with the transfer sanitisation procedures, prior to aseptic processing.

Sufficient space should be allowed around the working frontage to allow personnel to move in the room without disrupting the air flow in the cabinet. Typically this would be at least one metre. The movement of the operatives in the cabinet should be controlled to minimise the disturbance of air flow patterns.

7.6.1.3   Items should be placed in such a manner as to ensure minimal disruption to the air flow (see Chapter 10: Aseptic processing).

7.6.2   Pharmaceutical isolators

7.6.2.1   The design of the isolator should follow the principles laid down in *Isolators for Pharmaceutical Applications*. Guidance on the operating pressure in isolators for pharmaceutical use is provided (Midcalf et al 2014).

Consideration should always be given to installing a system of isolators which are gaseously biodecontaminated, in order to provide a high level of assurance of elimination of microbial contamination.

7.6.2.2   The critical zones of isolators that are used for the preparation of hazardous pharmaceuticals, e.g. cytotoxic drugs and radiopharmaceuticals, should operate at a negative pressure with respect to the background environment or be designed in such a way as to maximise operator protection as well as maintaining an appropriate level of product protection (HSE and MHRA 2015). 100Pa ± 20Pa is commonly used for positive and negative pressure isolators for pharmaceutical use.

7.6.2.3   Isolators used for handling hazardous pharmaceuticals should be totally exhausted to the outside environment, with appropriate safeguards (HSE and MHRA 2015).

The use of isolators compared to Class II Microbiological Safety Cabinets is preferable to maximise both operator and product protection.

7.6.2.4   Particular emphasis should be placed on ensuring that the glove/sleeve assembly or gauntlet maintains the integrity of the isolator during each and every session (see Chapter 11: Monitoring). Visual inspection of gloves and gauntlets forms an important part of the assessment of integrity but should not be relied upon alone. A pressure measuring device is often used, however its sensitivity should be determined during commissioning by applying different sized holes to a glove. Cabinet leak tests are a better indicator of the integrity of gloves.

7.6.2.5 The specified leak rate by pressure decay is a critical parameter that allows the user to assess whether its integrity has been compromised. Leak rates of 0.25% for negative isolators and 1% for positive isolators have been advocated (Coles 2012, Bässler 2013). This represents a drop of 25Pa in 6 minutes and 1.5 minutes respectively. A low leak rate is especially important for turbulent flow isolators. Ideally, the inner chamber should be leak tested separately from the whole carcass.

7.6.2.6 Transfer devices are designed so that they do not compromise the EU GMP Grade A (EC 2015) working zone during the transfer of materials and components. An input hatch door release timer should be specified with a minimum of 2 minutes to ensure adequate disinfection time and evaporation.

The transfer of materials and components into and out of the critical zone represents a significant challenge to the integrity of the isolator.

7.6.2.7 A service contract should be in place for all critical equipment (see Chapter 11: Monitoring).

7.6.3 Other equipment

7.6.3.1 The impact of other equipment, such as compounders, automated filling systems, radiopharmacy HPLC, dose calibrators etc. on disturbance of air flow in clean environments should be risk assessed (MHRA 2015).

7.7 Gowning

The operator is an essential part of the aseptic preparation process in hospitals. To minimise the risk of contaminating products with microorganisms and particles originating from the operators, it is essential to wear clean room clothing the quality of which should be appropriate for the process and the EU GMP grade of the working area (EC 2015).

7.7.1 A defined hand wash employing a biocidal agent should be used immediately before entering the aseptic suite. This should be followed by the routine application of a disinfectant hand rub/gel at the point of gloving.

Alcoholic gels and rubs are not appropriate for use on gloves as the emollients may damage glove materials; therefore alcohol 70% should be used.

7.7.2　The changing process should be defined and documented, and should include details of the appropriate clothing to be worn in each area.

7.7.3　The minimum requirement for clothing for each grade of environment is given in Table 7.1:

Table 7.1
Minimum clothing requirements

GRADE OF ENVIRONMENT	MINIMUM CLOTHING REQUIREMENTS
D	■ Hair, and where relevant, facial hair, beards and moustaches including stubble should be completely covered, for example with a beard snood ■ A non-shedding protective coat or suit ■ Dedicated shoes or overshoes.
C	■ Hair, and where relevant, facial hair, beards and moustaches including stubble should be completely covered, for example with a beard snood ■ A single- or two-piece trouser suit (which sheds virtually no fibres or particulate matter), gathered at the wrists and with a high neck ■ Dedicated shoes or overshoes.
B	■ Headgear should totally enclose hair, and where relevant, facial hair, beards and moustaches including stubble; it should be tucked into the neck of the suit ■ A sterile face mask ■ Non-powdered sterile gloves ■ A single piece clean room coverall, gathered at the wrists and with a high neck ■ Trouser legs should be tucked inside the footwear and garment sleeves into the gloves ■ Dedicated footwear, e.g. clean room slippers ■ All clothing should shed virtually no fibres or particulate matter and should be sterilised*.

7.7.4　The changing procedures should be appropriate for the grade of room specified and the processes undertaken.

7.7.5　On entering the clean room suite, unnecessary outdoor clothing and accessories should be removed and footwear should be changed or overshoes used.

7.7.6   Typical changing processes are indicated in Table 7.2:

Table 7.2
Typical changing processes

STAGE	GRADE D	GRADE C	GRADE B
1	Remove outdoor clothing and accessories	Remove outdoor clothing and accessories	Remove outdoor clothing and accessories
2	**Either** Don dedicated coat, hat and footwear (bare feet in clogs are not permitted) **or** Remove outer clothing down to underwear ■ tights and socks are acceptable – Don a dedicated ■ one or two piece suit ■ footwear (bare feet in clogs are not permitted – disposable clean room socks are preferred) ■ head covering ■ gloves Facial hair should be completely covered	Remove outer clothing down to underwear ■ tights and socks are acceptable – Don a dedicated ■ one or two piece suit ■ footwear (bare feet in clogs are not permitted – disposable clean room socks are preferred) ■ head covering ■ gloves Facial hair should be completely covered	Remove outer clothing down to underwear ■ tights and socks are acceptable – **Don a dedicated ■ one or two piece suit ■ footwear (bare feet in clogs are not permitted – disposable clean room socks are preferred) ■ head covering ■ gloves Facial hair should be completely covered
3			■ Don sterile* coverall, hood, mask, boots and gloves, over stage 2 clothing

* Sterilised clean room clothing should be worn by all staff entering the EU GMP Grade B (EC 2015) room. Alternative methods that guarantee the clothing is initially free from viable organisms may be used, e.g. a validated biocidal wash. Levels of particulate contamination should also be controlled.

** Specialised clean room undergarments are an acceptable alternative.

7.7.7   If the movement is from an EU GMP Grade D (EC 2015) support room to an EU GMP Grade D (EC 2015) isolator room, there should be a minimum of a change of gloves and footwear.

Best practice would be a change of footwear (or additional overshoes) and replacement of a coat. If a two piece suit is worn, an additional coat should be worn in the cleaner area.

7.7.8   There should be a periodic review of the garments and their fit to specifications (recommended annually).

The garment should be subject to validated laundering and, where appropriate, sterilisation processes. These processes should be subject to a regular audit.

7.7.9   There should be procedures in place detailing the use of garments and identifying the length of time they may be worn and how they are stored whilst not in use. Sterile garments for use in EU GMP Grade B (EC 2015) rooms should be worn for one session only.

7.7.10   The changing frequency for clean room coats for EU GMP Grade D (EC 2015) should not be less frequently than weekly, however changing frequency should be increased if the garment is worn for most of the working day.

References

Bässler HJ, Lehmann F (2013). *Containment Technology: Progress in the Pharmaceutical and Food Processing Industry.* London: Springer. p129.

Beaney AM, ed. (2010). *Design, Build and Maintenance of Pharmacy Aseptic Units.* 2nd edn. NHS Pharmaceutical Quality Assurance Committee.

British Standards Institute (BSI) (1999). *BS EN ISO 14644-1:1999 Clean Rooms and Associated Controlled Environments. Part 1: Classification of Air Cleanliness.* London: BSI.

Coles T (2012). Leak rate measurement for pharmaceutical isolators: Practical guidance for operators and test engineers. *Clean air and Containment Review.* Issue 11. 8-12.

Department of Health (DH) (2007). *Specialised ventilation for healthcare premises Part A: Design and validation heating and ventilation systems.* Health Technical Memorandum 03-01:2007. London: Department of Health.

Department of Health (DH) (2013). *Health Building Note 14-01 - Pharmacy and radiopharmacy facilities.* London: Department of Health.

European Association of Nuclear Medicine (EANM). Available at: ***http://www.eanm.org/publications/guidelines/5_EJNMMI_Guidance_cGRPPfulltext_05_2010.pdf*** (accessed 19 March 2016).

European Commission (2015). *The rules governing medicinal products in the European Community. Vol IV. Good Manufacturing Practice for medicinal products.* Available at: ***http://ec.europa.eu/health/documents/eudralex/vol-4/index_en.htm*** (accessed 26 February 2016).

Health and Safety Executive (HSE) and Medicines and Healthcare products Regulatory Agency (MHRA) (2015). *Handling cytotoxic drugs in isolators in NHS Pharmacies MS37.* Available at: ***www.hse.gov.uk/pubns/ms37.pdf*** (accessed 26 February 2016).

Institute of Physics and Engineering in Medicine (IPEM) (2011). *Medical Cyclotrons (including PET Radiopharmaceutical Production).* Report 105.

Medicines and Healthcare products Regulatory Agency (MHRA) (2015). *Questions and Answers for Specials Manufacturers.* London: MHRA. Available at: ***www.gov.uk/government/publications/guidance-for-specials-manufacturers*** (accessed 19 February 2016).

Midcalf B et al (2004). *Pharmaceutical Isolators.* London: Pharmaceutical Press.

Theobald A, ed (2011). *Sampson's Textbook of Radiopharmacy.* 4th edn. London: Pharmaceutical Press, 476-479.

UK Radiopharmacy Group (UKRG) (2009). *Guidelines for the safe preparation of radiolabelled blood cells.* Available at: ***http://www.bnms.org.uk/images/stories/downloads/documents/ukrg_blood_labelling_2009.pdf*** (accessed 26 February 2016).

UK Radiopharmacy Group (UKRG) and NHS Pharmaceutical Quality Assurance Committee (PQAC) (2012). *Quality Assurance of Radiopharmaceuticals.* Available at: ***www.bnms.org.uk/images/stories/UKRG/UKRG_QA_Apr-12.pdf*** (accessed 26 February 2016).

CHAPTER 8 PHARMACEUTICAL QUALITY SYSTEM

Developments in EU Good Manufacturing Practice (GMP) (EC 2015) have highlighted the need for a robust Pharmaceutical Quality System (PQS) (ICH 2008). Anyone preparing medicines should embrace the concept of Quality Management, that covers all matters, which individually or collectively influence the quality of the product.

Quality Management (previously Quality Assurance) is 'the sum total of the organised arrangements made with the objective of ensuring that medicinal products are of the quality required for their intended use'. Quality Management therefore incorporates GMP (EC 2015).

In accordance with EU GMP (EC 2015), senior managers have overall responsibility for the PQS and associated quality indicators (see Chapter 5: Management). It is, however, everyone's responsibility to comply with the quality system.

8.1   Pharmaceutical Quality System – general principles

8.1.1   A robust PQS should be in place incorporating EU GMP (EC 2015) and Quality Risk Management (ICH 2005).

8.1.2   The PQS should be fully documented, for example in a quality manual, and its effectiveness monitored.

8.1.3   Senior management should determine and provide adequate and appropriate resources (human, financial, materials, facilities and equipment) to implement and maintain the PQS and continually improve its effectiveness. They should ensure that resources are appropriately applied to a specific product, process or site. (See Chapter 5: Management.)

8.1.4   There should be defined Quality Management (previously Quality Assurance) duties specifically enshrined in job descriptions.

8.2   Design of the PQS

The design of the PQS should reflect the size and complexity of the preparation activities and should incorporate risk management principles (ICH 2005). It should, as a minimum, include the following:

8.2.1 Quality aspects throughout the product lifecycle

8.2.1.1 That is, product initiation, regular preparation, discontinuation (ICH 2008). There should be procedures in place for:

- Product initiation: This should consider, for example, risk assessments (see Chapter 3: Minimising risk with injectable medicines), formulation and stability (see Chapter 6: Formulation, stability and shelf life), change control
- Regular preparation: This should consider the impact on capacity of any increased frequency of preparation, review of trends etc.
- Product discontinuation: There should be a procedure to assess the impact of the discontinuation on patients, to consider alternative treatments, if appropriate, and to manage the discontinuation process.

8.2.2 Documentation control systems

8.2.2.1 In addition to the requirements in 8.3 below, there should be an overarching procedure that defines responsibility for writing, verifying and approving, and archiving, all types of documentation (SOPs, worksheets, specifications, logs etc).

8.2.3 Standard operating procedures

See section 8.4

8.2.4 Validation Master Plans

8.2.4.1 This includes computerised systems (see Part B – 2.6).

8.2.4.2 There should be a comprehensive and current Validation Master Plan (VMP) that summarises all validation activities carried out in the unit. Additionally, there may be individual VMPs for specific equipment or activities (PQAC 2009).

8.2.5 Deviation Management, planned and unplanned, e.g. deviations, microbiological non-conformances, error reporting, accident reporting, minor defect reporting systems

Note: Planned deviations may be more appropriately managed as temporary change controls.

8.2.5.1 There should be a suitable system, or series of systems, for management and trending of all types of deviations and sufficient resource to implement this in a timely manner.

8.2.5.2   Investigations of deviations should include an appropriate level of root cause analysis. Corrective and/or preventative actions (CAPAs) should be identified as a result of these investigations and their effectiveness should be monitored and assessed. Where human error is suspected as the cause, care should be taken to ensure that any process, procedural or system-based errors or problems have not been overlooked.

8.2.6   Change control

8.2.6.1   There should be a robust system for documenting and approving all planned changes (both temporary or permanent). All changes should be evaluated for their potential impact on product quality, and a decision made on whether or not to implement them.

8.2.6.2   Implementation of all changes should be tracked and they should be reviewed after a suitable period to ascertain whether they have worked as intended and to establish whether they have had any unanticipated detrimental impact on product quality.

8.2.7   Quality Review

8.2.7.1   There should be periodic management review, with the involvement of senior management, of the operation of the PQS to identify opportunities for continual improvement of products, processes and the system itself (see Chapter 5: Management).

8.2.8   Personnel and training policies (see Chapter 9: Personnel, training and competency assessment)

8.2.8.1   An approved and current training programme should be available. Completion of training should be documented in individual training records.

8.2.8.2   A system for the evaluation of the training programme, paying particular attention to practical skills, should be implemented (see Part B – 2.4).

8.2.9   Management of outsourced activities (see Chapter 5: Management)

8.2.9.1   Suitable technical agreements should be in place that define responsibilities for any outsourced activities and products. (A specimen technical agreement is given in Part B – 3).

8.2.9.2 Sufficient resource should be available to define and monitor technical agreements (see Chapter 3: Minimising risk with injectable medicines).

8.2.10 Internal audit (see Chapter 16: Internal and external audit)

8.2.10.1 A comprehensive programme of internal audits should be undertaken with the awareness and support of senior management, to review the continued effectiveness and further development of the PQS.

8.2.11 Complaints (see Chapter 15: Storage and distribution)

8.2.11.1 A system should be in place to record, investigate and identify the reason for any complaints.

8.2.11.2 Complaints should be closed out in a timely manner and reviewed regularly for trends as part of quality management meetings (see Chapter 5: Management).

8.2.12 Product recall (see Chapter 15: Storage and distribution)

8.2.12.1 There should be robust procedures for recall that are tested for efficiency and timeliness on an annual basis if an actual recall has not been undertaken.

8.3 Documentation – general issues

8.3.1 A comprehensive documentation system with clear detail should be in place. The Accountable Pharmacist has responsibility for the approval of all systems of work and documentation used in the unit. All documents should be independently approved.

8.3.2 Appropriate document controls should be in place i.e. unique identification, author, approved signatory, approval date, issue date and date for review, reference for superseded version.

8.3.3 In any one unit, worksheets and labels should have a standardised style and presentation within product type.

8.3.4 All documents should be regularly reviewed at defined intervals. Superseded documents should be clearly identified as such and should be retained for a sufficient period to satisfy legislative requirements. (East Anglia Medicines Information Service 2015).

8.3.5 Any draft documents should be identified and carefully controlled so that there is no risk that an incorrect version could be inadvertently approved for use.

8.4 Standard operating procedures

Standard operating procedures should be written in clear, numbered steps in the imperative tense and should include the following:

- control of documentation systems
- deviation management
- change control
- receipt of orders, including prescription verification and transcription
- purchasing, receipt and storage of components
- cleaning, disinfection and sanitation processes
- entering and exiting from clean areas, including the correct use of protective clothing
- environmental monitoring (both physical and microbiological) of the clean rooms and clean air devices
- use of any equipment required for preparation, including cleaning and calibration instructions where appropriate
- generation of worksheets and labels
- product preparation, checking and release
- process validation, including media fills
- staff training, including operator validation using broth transfer trials and formal skills assessment
- actions to be taken when failures are identified by the monitoring systems, e.g. process simulations or operator validation tests, environmental monitoring and sterility tests
- storage and distribution
- product complaints and recalls, and handling of defective products (including, where appropriate, a defect log)
- product returns.

8.5 Worksheets

8.5.1 Individual worksheets reproduced from a suitably approved master format should be used, including electronic formats.

8.5.2 The worksheet should be sufficiently detailed to allow the traceability of starting materials and components, where appropriate, to establish an audit trail for the product (see Chapter 13: Starting materials, components and consumables).

8.5.3 Completed worksheets should be retained for a sufficient period to satisfy legislative requirements. (East Anglia Medicines Information Service 2015).

8.5.4 Worksheets will vary for each unit and should be designed to promote good workflow and to minimise the possibility of transcription errors. They should include:

- the name and/or formula of the product
- a unique identifier for the product
- a written protocol for routinely-prepared products
- manufacturers and batch numbers of medicinal ingredients, listed in order of the compounding process where the order of mixing is important e.g. manual additions to parenteral nutrition solutions
- manufacturers and batch numbers of sterile components used to prepare the product, where appropriate (see Chapter 13: Starting materials, components and consumables)
- date of preparation
- expiry date and time (if applicable) of product
- the signature or initials of staff carrying out preparation and checking procedures
- details of any calculation and the signature or initials of staff carrying out and independently checking such calculations
- the signature or initials of the Authorised Pharmacist or Accredited Product Approver releasing the product, and the date of approval
- a label reconciliation procedure for all labels
- a record of the label on the product
- the patient's name (or other identifier)
- the patient's age for paediatric patients (aged under 16) to the nearest year or nearest month if under 1 year, where systems allow for this (Toft 2012)
- a comments section for recording any unusual occurrences, deviations, or observations.

8.5.5 There should be clear differentiation of paediatric worksheets. The use of colour should be considered (Toft 2012).

8.6 Other documentation

8.6.1 Operation, cleaning, maintenance and fault logs should be kept for all facilities and equipment. All planned preventative maintenance and breakdown maintenance should be recorded for key equipment and facilities.

8.6.2 A planned deviation (temporary change control) form should be available for all products made outside the standard operational procedures. Where deviations from specifications occur, measures taken to ensure that the final product is satisfactory should be documented.

8.6.3 A record should be maintained of errors and near-misses and of investigations undertaken. Trending should be carried out.

8.6.4 Units should participate in the Pharmaceutical Aseptic Services Group (PASG), national aseptic error monitoring scheme, or the UK Radiopharmacy Group error reporting scheme (if appropriate).

8.6.5 Risk analysis, trending and corrective and/or preventative actions (CAPA) should be carried out to an appropriate level depending upon severity.

8.6.6 There should be a record of the Authorised Pharmacist supervising each preparation session.

8.7 Computerised systems (see also Part B – 2.6)

8.7.1 Where computerised systems are in use, access should be restricted, by use of passwords or similar, to staff trained to use the system, with records being retained of any such training.

8.7.2 If a computerised system is used for document control, the system should be fully validated using a risk-based approach to decide the level of validation required. In such cases, the computerised system should demonstrate a level of accuracy and traceability which is at least as good as any paper-based system it replaces.

8.7.3 If document masters are held electronically, there should be a demonstrable system of backups of the master copies. In addition, there should be a failsafe or fallback system in place to allow timely provision of up-to-date documents in the event of computerised system failure.

8.7.4   Where an electronic prescribing system is linked to the generation of an electronic worksheet, patient details, doses etc. should be verified initially and checked manually at the product approval stage against the prescription (see Chapter 4: Prescribing, clinical pharmacy and aseptic services verification, and Chapter 14: Product approval).

8.7.5   Planned updates or alterations to a validated computerised system should be handled via a formal change control process employing a risk-based impact assessment of the proposed changes to hardware or software.

8.7.6   Periodic rolling re-validation is recommended for critical computerised systems at regular intervals (suggested every three years) to ensure maintenance of a validated state. If this is not the case, a written justification should be on file.

8.7.7   Records held solely in electronic form should remain accessible for the life of the document. Where this period exceeds the working life of the system, provision should be made for retaining access to records in a timely fashion.

8.7.8   Where a computerised system fulfills a critical function in the aseptic process, there should be a robust back-up system in place, which allows continued use of the system in the event of hardware, software or network failure. The procedure for switching to the back-up should be documented and periodically tested.

8.8   Labels

8.8.1   Labels should comply with all statutory and professional requirements including the *British Pharmacopoeia* monograph on Unlicensed Medicines. (BP Commission Secretariat, current edition).

8.8.2   Labels should be clear, unambiguous, with no overtyping of content during generation.

8.8.3   They should include the following information:

- approved name of medicine (brand name for biologicals)
- quantity and strength
- vehicle containing the drug when used as a diluent
- final volume
- route of administration
- expiry date and time (if applicable)

■ batch number (or other unique identifier)

■ appropriate cautionary notices

■ storage requirements

■ name of patient (or other identifier)

■ name and address of pharmacy.

The following may also be included:

■ preparation date

■ patient's location

■ rate of administration, e.g. for parenteral nutrition

■ patient's hospital number

■ Controlled Drug (if applicable).

Note: POM should not be stated on the label for an unlicensed medicine.

8.8.4 For parenteral nutrition, the maximum concentration of Glucose or osmolarity that can be infused peripherally should be agreed locally and any solutions containing in excess of this concentration should be labelled 'To be given by central line only' (DH 2011).

8.8.5 Vinca alkaloids should be labelled 'Fatal if given by any other route' (NPSA 2008).

8.8.6 Intrathecal products should be labelled 'For intrathecal use only' (DH 2008).

References

British Pharmacopoeia Commission Secretariat. *British Pharmacopoeia*. Current edn. London: The Stationery Office.

Department of Health (DH) (2008). *Updated National Guidance on Safe Administration of Intrathecal Chemotherapy*. HSC 2008/001. London: Department of Health.

Department of Health (DH) (2011). *Improving practice and reducing risk in the provision of parenteral nutrition for neonates and children*. Report from the Paediatric Chief Pharmacists Group. London: Department of Health. Available at: **www.rpharms.com** (accessed 04 April 2016).

East Anglia Medicines Information Service (2015). *Recommendations for the Retention of Pharmacy Records*. v5. Available at: **www.medicinesresources.nhs.uk/en/Communities/NHS/SPS-E-and-SE-England/Reports-Bulletins/Retention-of-pharmacy-records** (accessed on 06 April 2016).

European Commission (2015). *The rules governing medicinal products in the European Community. Vol IV. Good Manufacturing Practice for medicinal products*. Available at: **http://ec.europa.eu/health/documents/eudralex/vol-4/index_en.htm** (accessed 26 February 2016).

International Conference on Harmonisation of Technical Requirements for Registration of Pharmaceuticals for Human Use (ICH) (2005). *Harmonised Tripartite Guideline, Quality Risk Management, Q9*. Available at: **www.ich.org/fileadmin/Public_Web_Site/ICH_Products/Guidelines/Quality/Q9/Step4/Q9_Guideline.pdf** (accessed 04 April 2016).

International Conference on Harmonisation of Technical Requirements for Registration of Pharmaceuticals for Human Use (ICH) (2008). *Harmonised Tripartite Guideline, Pharmaceutical Quality System, Q10*.

National Patient Safety Agency (NPSA) (2008). *Rapid Response Report. Using Vinca Alkaloid Minibags (Adult/ Adolescent Units)* NPSA/2008/RRR004. Available at: **www.nrls.npsa.nhs.uk/alerts/?entryid45=59890&p=2** (accessed 26 February 2016).

NHS Pharmaceutical Quality Assurance Committee (PQAC) (2009). *Validation Master Plans*. Edition 1.

Pharmaceutical Aseptic Services Group (PASG) **www.pasg.nhs.uk**

Toft B (2012). *Independent review of the circumstances surrounding a serious untoward incident that occurred in the Aseptic Manufacturing Unit, Royal Surrey County Hospital on Monday, 18 June 2012*. Available at: **www.chfg.org/wp-content/uploads/2013/01/Report-to-medical-Director-RSCH_ProfBToft.pdf** (accessed 06 April 2016).

QUALITY ASSURANCE OF ASEPTIC PREPARATION SERVICES:
STANDARDS HANDBOOK PART A

CHAPTER 9 PERSONNEL, TRAINING AND COMPETENCY ASSESSMENT

It is essential for individuals to demonstrate their competence and for organisations to accurately and appropriately record training and competence of staff for the role or task they are undertaking.

Use should be made of appropriate resources such as those on the NHS TSET, GPhC, RPS and Skills for Health websites to support individuals and organisations meet these operational standards and also provide support for more advanced roles.

9.1 Personnel

9.1.1 Any aseptic preparation service should be managed by an Accountable Pharmacist who has current practical and theoretical experience in aseptic preparation and/or manufacture. (At least two years' experience in an aseptic unit would normally be expected.) A pharmacist working in a locum capacity is not normally acceptable to perform an Accountable Pharmacist role. The Accountable Pharmacist should be knowledgeable in all aspects of aseptic preparation, including the following areas:

- Good Manufacturing Practice (GMP) as defined by EU GMP (EC 2015)
- formulation
- validation
- aseptic processing
- pharmaceutical quality systems (PQS)
- quality control
- radiopharmacy and radiation protection (where applicable).

9.1.2 The Accountable Pharmacist should have this title and associated responsibilities clearly stated in their job description.

9.1.3 The Accountable Pharmacist should be assured that the facilities and systems in place are capable, on a day-to-day basis, of providing an adequate quality service able to meet the needs of patients.

QUALITY ASSURANCE OF ASEPTIC PREPARATION SERVICES:
STANDARDS HANDBOOK PART A

9.1.4 Any Authorised Pharmacist called on to deputise for the Accountable Pharmacist should have the necessary level of training and knowledge, and be clear about the limits of his/her authority and responsibility in this deputising role. These limits should be agreed with the Accountable Pharmacist.

9.1.5 Specific aspects of the service can be delegated to an Accredited Product Approver provided that they are given clear and precise training in both his/her duties and the limits of authority and responsibility are defined.

9.1.6 Before undertaking radiopharmacy preparation, staff are required to achieve 'adequate training' as defined (IR(ME)R 2000).

9.1.7 Anyone entering the unit that is not involved in the aseptic preparation process, e.g. staff, service engineers and visitors, should observe the rules on clothing applicable for the area. (A simplified training procedure on the elements of GMP for personnel entering the clean room facility, e.g. engineers and cleaning staff, should also be available and they should be observed where possible.)

9.2 Staff hygiene

9.2.1 Standards of hygiene are of critical importance in aseptic processing and staff should maintain high standards of personal hygiene. This should be detailed locally in a standard operating procedure.

9.2.2 Staff should be required to report skin lesions, known infections or potential symptoms of infections to the Authorised Pharmacist supervising at the time. A decision should be made as to whether staff carry out the full range of duties under these circumstances.

9.2.3 Within an aseptic unit, GMP overrides religious practices for patient safety reasons. Suitably designed clean room clothing may be acceptable from both GMP and religious perspectives and should be sought, if appropriate.

9.2.4 Tattoos and piercings should be managed in the same way as skin lesions in the Occupational Health policy. This will normally mean that personnel will be excluded from clean areas until any tattoo or piercing has healed.

9.2.5 Wrist watches and jewellery should not be worn. Piercings, if not removed, should be covered.

9.2.6 Cosmetics, nail varnish, false nails, false eyelashes etc., should not be worn in clean areas.

9.3 Training

9.3.1 All staff should receive training and be assessed as competent for the range of activities they will perform in their role, as outlined in recognised competency frameworks such as those from NHS TSET, RPS, Skills for Health etc. Training should provide staff with at least:

- an appropriate knowledge of current EU GMP (EC 2015)
- a knowledge of local practices, including health and safety
- a knowledge of pharmaceutical microbiology
- a working knowledge of the department, products and services provided.

9.3.2 An approved and current training programme should be available. Completion of training should be documented in individual training records. A system for the evaluation of the training programme, paying particular attention to practical skills, should be implemented (see Part B – 2.4).

9.3.3 An individual training record should be available for each member of staff. This should include the following:

- current job description
- initial training (may include hospital specific mandatory requirements, e.g. infection control)
- operator validation
- external training courses
- in-house GMP training
- additional training, e.g. competency assessment/logs etc.

9.4 Competency assessment

9.4.1 Initial training should involve competency assessment and sign off at appropriate levels.

9.4.2 Regular reassessment of the competency of each member of staff should be undertaken, and revision or retraining provided where necessary.

9.4.3 The effectiveness of any additional training or retraining needed as a result of a deficiency should be checked after delivery and after a further time interval to ensure that the additional training has been effective and is retained.

9.4.4   A key element of operator competency is regular assessment of aseptic technique using broth. (The recommended procedure is referred to in Part B – 2.2.) This should be complemented by regular observation of aseptic technique to ensure that the operator can prepare dosage units precisely and safely.

9.4.5   Initial competence of operators should be established by the successful completion of three consecutive Universal Operator Broth Transfer Validation Tests. Regular re-assessment (at least six-monthly) should be undertaken. In the event of failure, an investigation should be undertaken and three consecutive operator broth transfer validation tests should be successfully undertaken.

9.4.6   Another key element is the demonstration of competency to perform calculations correctly for the tasks being undertaken (Toft B 2012).

9.4.7   Any staff undertaking checking should have evidence that they are competent to do so. Use should be made of national competency frameworks (ASAWG 2014).

9.4.8   Where a suitably trained member of staff has been absent from the aseptic operation for more than 6 months, the Accountable Pharmacist should assure him/herself as to the competence of that member of staff before allowing him/her to resume aseptic preparation.

9.4.9   There should be a commitment to a programme of development for all staff. Use should be made of the Technical Professional Development Portal (**www.tpdportal.org.uk**) when appropriate.

References

General Pharmaceutical Council (GPhC). Minimum training requirements for dispensing/pharmacy assistants. Available at: **http://www.pharmacyregulation.org/education/support-staff/dispensing-assistant** (accessed 25 February 2016).

NHS Aseptic Services Accreditations Working Group (ASAWG) (2014). *Nationally Recognised Competency Framework for Pharmacists and Pharmacy Technicians: Product Approval (Release) in Aseptic Services under Section 10 Exemption.* Available at: **www.nhspedc.nhs.uk/supports.htm** (accessed 25 February 2016).

NHS Technical Specialist Education and Training (TSET). Technical Professional Development (TPD) Portal. Available at: **www.tpdportal.org.uk** (accessed 25 February 2016).

NHS Technical Specialist Education and Training (TSET) Aseptic Processing Program. Available at: **www.tset.org.uk** (accessed 25 February 2016).

Royal Pharmaceutical Society (RPS) Faculty. Available at **www.rpharms.com/faculty** (accessed 05 April 2016).

Skills for Health National Occupational Standards. Available at: **http://tools.skillsforhealth.org.uk/** (accessed 25 February 2016).

The Ionising Radiation (Medical Exposure) Regulations (IR(ME)R) 2000. SI 2000 No. 1059. London: The Stationery Office.

Toft B (2012). *Independent review of the circumstances surrounding a serious untoward incident that occurred in the Aseptic Manufacturing Unit, Royal Surrey County Hospital on Monday, 18 June 2012.* Available at: **www.chfg.org/wp-content/uploads/2013/01/Report-to-medical-Director-RSCH_ProfBToft.pdf** (accessed 06 April 2016).

CHAPTER 10 ASEPTIC PROCESSING

When sterile products are manipulated aseptically there is always a risk that microbial contamination may occur. A high level of sterility assurance can be achieved by:

- good clean room design (see Chapter 7: Facilities and equipment)
- good process design
- comprehensive validation of the facility, equipment, and the preparation processes

- control of starting materials and components (see Chapter 13: Starting materials, components and consumables)
- control of the aseptic processes e.g. by use of standard operating procedures, monitoring, training, competency assessment, supervision, etc.

10.1 Process design

In designing the process, consideration should be given to risks from microbial contamination (see Chapter 3: Minimising risk with injectable medicines), risks of errors in preparation (e.g. wrong drug or wrong volume, cross contamination of products, particulate contamination) and risks to the staff involved in the preparation (e.g. exposure to hazardous substances, injuries from sharps or repetitive strain injuries). There may also be additional considerations for gaseous biodecontamination isolators and for radiopharmacy for radiation protection.

10.1.1 Entry and exit of personnel, gowning and gloving

10.1.1.1 Changing and washing procedures should be designed to minimise contamination of clean area clothing or carry through of contaminants to the clean areas.

10.1.1.2 Clean room clothing should be appropriate to the grade of the working area and changed at appropriate frequency (see Chapter 7: Facilities and equipment).

10.1.1.3 Wrist watches, cosmetics and jewellery should not be worn in clean areas (see Chapter 9: Personnel, training and competency assessment).

10.1.1.4   Exit procedures should ensure safe and appropriate disposal of waste (DH 2013) removal and disposal/segregation of gloves and clean room clothing and hand washing to prevent cross contamination or inadvertent exposure to hazardous substances (COSHH 2002).

10.1.2 Choice of equipment and materials

10.1.2.1   The clean air device to be used for aseptic preparation should be selected based on product type, equipment availability and relative risks of microbial contamination and risks to operators (e.g. potential exposure to hazardous substances or ergonomic issues).

10.1.2.2   Triple- or double-wrapped, sterile disposable equipment should be used where available to avoid or reduce the need for disinfection of the outer surface during transfer.

10.1.2.3   Vials should be used, where possible, in preference to ampoules, as this better enables the maintenance of a 'closed procedure' for aseptic compounding.

10.1.2.4   Aseptic preparation processes should be designed to minimise the use of sharps. (*The Health and Safety (Sharp Instruments in Healthcare) Regulations 2013*). Only if non-sharp or safer-sharp devices are not available or reasonably practical should exposed sharps be used. Re-sheathing of needles by hand after use is not permitted. If re-sheathing is undertaken (e.g. for radiation protection reasons in radiopharmacy) this should be documented in a risk assessment and safe working practices implemented to reduce risk of injury (UKRG 2013, PASG 2014).

10.1.3 Good aseptic practice principles

10.1.3.1   Aseptic preparation processes should be designed to minimise the number of aseptic connections/manipulations. A summary table covering all the products prepared (grouping of similar products is acceptable) and the typical maximum number of aseptic connections/manipulations with any relevant comments should be available on file.

10.1.3.2   Closed procedures should be used (as this is one of the conditions for aseptic preparation in an unlicensed unit).

10.1.3.3 All materials transferred into the clean room and critical zone should be sanitised prior to transfer (see Chapter 12: Cleaning, sanitisation and biodecontamination).

10.1.3.4 Syringes or needles packed in strips should be separated before transfer into the critical zone to reduce the potential for particle dispersion.

10.1.3.5 Starting materials transferred into the critical zone should be allowed to dry before proceeding with the preparation.

10.1.3.6 The critical zone should be kept free and uncluttered with any materials positioned in the critical zone so that there is unobstructed air flow over and around them. Materials should not be stored in the critical zone.

10.1.3.7 Operators should avoid reaching over the product to access equipment or dispose of waste.

10.1.3.8 Aseptic processing techniques used during manipulation of the product should ensure 'no-touch' of critical surfaces to avoid any contact with any surface which will be in contact with the sterile fluid path.

10.1.3.9 Over-wrapped items should be peeled open in the air stream from the HEPA filter in a manner that will minimise shedding of particles. Paper-backed items should not be torn open.

10.1.3.10 If re-sheathing of needles is required for containment or asepsis, a re-sheathing aid such as a needle block should be used (see 10.1.2.4).

10.1.3.11 The surfaces of bungs that will be penetrated and the necks of ampoules to be opened should be wiped with a fresh sterile 70% alcohol impregnated wipe and allowed to dry before proceeding.

10.1.3.12 Ampoules should be opened in the air stream from the HEPA filter.

10.1.3.13 When withdrawing from glass ampoules, a sterile filter straw or filter needle should be used to remove glass particles. The filter straw or needle should be replaced with a fresh sterile needle before adding the solution to another container. Alternatively the solution from an ampoule should be passed through a suitable filter into the final container so that any particles generated from the opening of the ampoule and extraction of liquid are removed.

10.1.3.14 Ampoules should only ever be used for a single withdrawal immediately after opening and then discarded (see Chapter 2 definition of closed procedure). If multiple ampoules are used, the withdrawal should be made before opening the next ampoule.

10.1.3.15 When using vials, pressure equalisation techniques using the syringe or venting devices should be employed to avoid aerosols.
Note: This may not be applicable in radiopharmacy.

10.1.3.16 When making additions to infusion bags, the additive port should be positioned so it is in the HEPA filtered air stream rather than on the work surface.

Best practice is to ensure that, wherever possible, manipulations are undertaken in mid-air, well away from work surfaces or other objects. Air flows more slowly close to surfaces increasing the chance of deposition of particles.

10.1.3.17 An appropriate gauge of needle should be used that will minimise damage to rubber bungs whilst still maintaining an acceptable flow rate.

10.1.3.18 Needles should be inserted through the centre of the additive port, keeping the needle straight to avoid puncturing the bag.

10.1.3.19 All tubing should be clear of fluid and securely clamped before removal from the critical zone.

10.1.3.20 The work surface and gloves should be sanitised between products or contacts during preparation activity. Time to allow drying after sanitisation is required.

10.1.3.21 Any spillage of product should be wiped up immediately. Gloves should be changed and the work surface cleaned and sanitised before continuing work. Consideration should be given to performing an additional set of finger dabs before changing gloves.

10.1.4 Product segregation and in-process checks

10.1.4.1 Processes should be designed with appropriate segregation of products and flow of materials to ensure there is no inadvertent cross contamination or mix-up of products.

10.1.4.2 Appropriate pre- and in-process checks required should be defined for each product type and suitably recorded (see Chapter 8: Pharmaceutical Quality System).

10.1.4.3 If vials are used for more than one patient (vial sharing) then it should be carried out on a campaign basis and there should be measures in place to ensure that there is a robust in-process checking system carried out by accredited in-process checkers (see Chapter 9: Personnel, training and competency assessment) including the drug, concentration and volume measured, unless all measurements can be checked retrospectively, i.e. the product is a liquid medicine solely drawn up into syringes which can then be volume checked at the product approval stage (PQAC 2014).

10.1.4.4 If auto-compounders are used (e.g. for parenteral nutrition preparation) checks on the correctness of set-up should include (MHRA 2015):

- The correct starting material is connected to the correct line. This check should be independent of set-up, and may be either a second operator or automated verification (e.g. barcode linking). Replenishment of starting solutions throughout the process should be similarly verified
- Volume delivery checks
- Independent check on the required volume for each solution
- Reconciliation of starting solutions at the end of the session
- Details of remaining manual additions.

10.1.4.5 Waste disposal procedures should be designed to prevent cross contamination and risks to personnel from hazardous substances or sharps and be in accordance with healthcare waste standards (DH 2013).

10.2 Validation

Validation of the aseptic process can be spilt into three distinct areas:

- Facility and equipment validation (see Chapter 7: Facilities and equipment)
- Process validation (see Part B – 2.1)
- Operator validation (see Part B – 2.2).

Validation should be performed when an aseptic unit is commissioned and when any new equipment, process, technique or member of staff is introduced into the process and at defined intervals. The purpose is to show that under simulated conditions aseptic products can be consistently prepared to the required quality using the defined process.

Any subsequent changes should be assessed in the same manner to ensure that they do not compromise that quality (see Chapter 8: Pharmaceutical Quality System).

Validation methods are described in more detail in Part B – 2 but it should be remembered that they only represent the capabilities of the aseptic processing system as tested. To ensure the reproducibility of quality of the product, strict adherence to the validated standard operating procedures is essential.

10.2.1 Process validations should be designed to cover the range of processes used within the unit and should reflect worst case (see 10.1.3.1).

10.2.2 Operator validations should be up to date and should cover the range of aseptic techniques and clean air devices which an operator will use.

10.3 Control of the aseptic process

10.3.1 All key elements and manipulative steps in the aseptic process, from the starting material to the finished product, should be controlled by comprehensive standard operating procedures to ensure that the process consistently produces a product of the requisite quality.

10.3.2 Aseptic processing should be carried out by validated staff (see 10.2).

10.3.3 Staff should be fully conversant with all the relevant standard operating procedures (as determined by their role) before being deemed competent to work in the aseptic preparation unit.

10.3.4 Regular updating of staff on the procedures should be undertaken, documented and the extent of knowledge assessed.

10.3.5 Pre- and in-process checking should be performed by appropriately accredited staff (see Chapter 9: Personnel, training and competency assessment).

10.3.6 All staff working in aseptic processing should be made fully aware of the potential consequences of any deviation from the validated procedure, both to the integrity of the product and to the intended recipient. Regular reminders of the critical nature of the process should be provided. Staff should report any unusual or unexpected occurrence and any errors they have, or might have, made to the Authorised Pharmacist supervising at the time (even if they have been immediately corrected). Any deviation should be fully documented and managed (see Chapter 8: Pharmaceutical Quality System).

10.3.7 There should be a formal system for the assessment of any proposed change which may affect product quality (see Chapter 8: Pharmaceutical Quality System).

10.3.8 Staff involved in aseptic processing should be taught to recognise upper limb disorders (repetitive strain injuries) and to use techniques to minimise these conditions wherever possible (PASG 1998).

10.3.9 Standard operating procedures should be written and implemented for all equipment used for aseptic processing (see Chapter 8: Pharmaceutical Quality System).

References

Department of Health (DH) (2013). *Safe management of healthcare waste*. Health Technical Memorandum 07-01. London: Department of Health.

Medicines and Healthcare products Regulatory Agency (MHRA) (2015). *Questions and Answers for Specials Manufacturers*. London: MHRA. Available at: *www.gov.uk/government/publications/guidance-for-specials-manufacturers* (accessed 19 February 2016).

NHS Pharmaceutical Aseptic Services Group (PASG) (1998). ULDs and You. *Repetitive Procedures in Aseptic Pharmacy Practice*. NHS Pharmaceutical Aseptic Services Group. Available at: *http://pasg.nhs.uk/documents.php?sid=46&sgid=33* (accessed 13 May 2016).

NHS Pharmaceutical Aseptic Services Group (PASG) (2014). *Guidance on Implementing the Health and Safety (Sharp Instruments in Healthcare) Regulations 2013 in NHS Pharmacy Aseptic Services*. NHS Pharmaceutical Aseptic Services Group. Available at: *http://pasg.nhs.uk/documents.php?sid=32&sgid=24* (accessed 13 May 2016).

NHS Pharmaceutical Quality Assurance Committee (PQAC) (2014). *Vial Sharing in Aseptic Services*. NHS Pharmaceutical Quality Assurance Committee. Available at: *www.medicinesresources.nhs.uk/en/Communities/NHS/UKQAInfoZone/National-resources/NHSPQA-Committee-/NHSPQA-Yellow-Cover-Guidance/Vial-Sharing-in-Aseptic-Services-Edition-1-August-2014/* (accessed 02 September 2015).

The Control of Substances Hazardous to Health Regulations (COSHH) 2002. SI 2002 No. 2677. London: The Stationery Office *www.legislation.gov.uk/uksi/2002/2677/pdfs/uksi_20022677_en.pdf* (accessed 04 February 2016).

The Health and Safety (Sharp Instruments in Healthcare) Regulations 2013. SI 2013 No. 645. London: The Stationery Office. Available at: *http://www.legislation.gov.uk/uksi/2013/645/made#f00002* (accessed 06 April 2016).

UK Radiopharmacy Group (UKRG) (2013). *Guidance on the recapping of needles in radiopharmacy and nuclear medicine*. Available at: *http://www.bnms.org.uk/images/Recapping_needles_UKRG_guidance_v5_UKRG_format.pdf* (accessed 26 February 2016).

CHAPTER 11 MONITORING

It is essential to ensure facilities and conditions are maintained and processes are followed in a consistent manner by all staff. This is ensured by regular monitoring and testing of the environment, process and finished product and forms an essential part of the quality assurance of all aseptically-prepared products. Standards and guidelines are available for many of the physical and microbiological aspects (Farwell 1995, EC 2015, BSI 1999b, BSI 2015, Midcalf et al 2004, PHSS 2002, PDA 1980, Needle and Sizer 1998, BSI 2000, UKRG 2012). The Accountable Pharmacist, Authorised Pharmacists and senior staff should refer to, and have an understanding of, these documents, with particular emphasis on the sections relating to aseptic processing.

Particular importance should be attached to obtaining meaningful results, monitoring trends, setting 'in-house' standards and action limits, investigating out-of-specification results and deviations and undertaking corrective and/or preventative actions (CAPA). Information should be actively and knowledgeably assessed and not merely filed for record purposes.

The monitoring programme forms an important part of the Pharmaceutical Quality System and comprises a programme of environmental monitoring carried out by the staff undertaking aseptic preparation and a series of planned preventative maintenance (PPM) and environmental tests undertaken by suitably trained personnel or contracted out to an appropriate organisation with an appropriate service level agreement and technical agreement (see Part B – 3).

11.1 Programme of monitoring and testing

11.1.1 Each unit should have a sessional, daily, weekly, monthly monitoring programme and a quarterly and annual testing programme. All results should be documented and retained for inspection.

A recommended frequency is shown for guidance in Tables 11.1 and 11.2. This should be considered to be a minimum requirement. The optimum frequency of testing will be a function of the individual unit and the activity within the unit. The programme should be such that it confirms that control of the environment within standards is maintained. It is not a substitute for the continual vigilance of operators in ensuring the correct functioning of all equipment. Rapid gaseous biodecontamination isolators are available for aseptic preparation and the frequency of testing could be reduced to the minimum frequency as in Table 11.1 if full confidence is established (Hiom et al 2004). However, any microbiological growth found should be considered as requiring a full investigation. (PICS 2007).

Table 11.1
Microbiological monitoring programme (minimum frequency)

TEST	LIQUID SANITISATION CRITICAL ZONE *	GASEOUS BIODECONTAMINATION CRITICAL ZONE **	CLEAN ROOM SUITE
Finger dabs	Sessional	Weekly	Not applicable
Settle plates	Sessional	Weekly	Weekly
Surface contact plates	Weekly	Weekly	Weekly
Active air samples	3 Monthly	3 Monthly	3 Monthly
Surface swabs ***	3 Monthly	3 Monthly	3 Monthly

* Liquid sanitisation includes wipe and spray into conventional isolators and cabinets.
** Gaseous biodecontamination includes VHP isolators.
*** Tests on equipment, uneven surfaces and crevices etc.

CHAPTER 11 MONITORING

Table 11.2.1
Physical monitoring programme of a clean room

ASEPTIC FACILITY TEST	MINIMUM FREQUENCY
Pressure differential between rooms	Monitor continuously, record daily
Pressure differential across HEPAs	Monitor continuously, record weekly
Particle counts	3 Monthly in use, annual 'at rest' – (MHRA 2015)
Air changes/hour	3 Monthly
Filter integrity/Installation leak test	Annual
Air flow pattern	Annual – EU GMP Grade B (EC 2015) or after significant work on the Air Handling Unit
Temperature of fridges	Monitor continuously, record daily
Temperature in critical storage rooms	Monitor continuously, record daily
Relative humidity *	Annual
Noise	Annual
Light	Annual
Clean up rate	After in use test

* *Relative humidity is a useful indicator of potential moisture condensation that could promote the growth of microbes and therefore 3 monthly measurement is advised.*

Table 11.2.2
Physical monitoring programme for a unidirectional air flow cabinet

UNIDIRECTIONAL AIR FLOW CABINET TEST	MINIMUM FREQUENCY
Pressure differential across HEPA	Monitor continuously, record daily
Particle counts	3 Monthly in use, annual 'at rest' – (MHRA 2015)
Air velocity	3 Monthly
Uniformity of air flow +/- 20%	3 Monthly
Filter integrity/Installation leak test	Annual*
Air flow pattern	Annual or after moving the cabinet
Noise	Annual
Light	Annual

* The MHRA (MHRA 2015) state a minimum of annually but early detection of a problem will reduce the risk of compromising the work area and a more frequent test schedule may be considered appropriate.

Table 11.2.3
Physical monitoring programme for a class 2 safety cabinet

CLASS 2 SAFETY CABINET TEST (BSI 2000)	MINIMUM FREQUENCY
Pressure differential of extract	Monitor continuously, record daily
Pressure differential across downflow HEPA	Monitor continuously, record daily
Particle counts	3 Monthly in use, annual 'at rest' – (MHRA 2015)
Air velocity	3 Monthly
Air uniformity +/- 20%	3 Monthly
Filter integrity/Installation leak test	Annual*
Product protection test**	Annual
Operator protection test***	Annual
Air flow pattern	Annual
Alarm function	Weekly
Noise	Annual
Light	Annual

* The MHRA (MHRA 2015) state a minimum of annually but early detection of a problem will reduce the risk of compromising the work area and a more frequent test schedule may be considered appropriate.

** The product protection test is considered to be desirable using appropriate methodology e.g. smoke and particle counts, external KI discus test (BSI 2000). Air inflow tests are not considered adequate.

*** This test is not essential in radiopharmacy as other operator protection testing is used, e.g. film badges.

QUALITY ASSURANCE OF ASEPTIC PREPARATION SERVICES:
STANDARDS HANDBOOK PART A

Table 11.2.4
Physical monitoring programme for isolators

ISOLATOR TEST	MINIMUM CHAMBER FREQUENCY	MINIMUM HATCH FREQUENCY
Pressure differential from chamber to external room	Monitor continuously if possible, record daily	Record weekly if possible
Pressure differential across HEPAs	Monitor continuously if possible, record daily	Record weekly if possible
Air changes per hour	Monitor continuously, record daily if measured	Record weekly if measured
Particle counts	3 Monthly in use, annual 'at rest' – (MHRA 2015)	Annual 'at rest'
Air velocity	3 Monthly	3 Monthly
Air uniformity – unless turbulent	3 Monthly	Not applicable
Filter integrity/Installation leak test	Annual*	Annual*
Glove/sleeve and gauntlet integrity	Sessional	Not applicable
Isolator leak test	-ve pressure weekly, +ve pressure monthly	-ve pressure weekly, +ve pressure monthly
Air flow pattern	Annual	Not applicable
Alarm function	Weekly	Not applicable
Door/hatch timer	Not applicable	Annual
Noise	Annual	Not applicable
Light	Annual	Not applicable

*The MHRA (MHRA 2015) state a minimum of annually but early detection of a problem will reduce the risk of compromising the work area and a more frequent test schedule may be considered appropriate.

11.1.2 Action and alert levels should be set to indicate when corrective action and investigation respectively should be carried out.

A monthly and annual review of trends and types of microorganisms should be made.

Trend data should be carried out for each workstation, operator, person carrying out the liquid sanitisation of items taken into the work area and for each clean room. (Species level identification of organisms can be of assistance when reviewing the effect of personnel on the clean room environment). (See Part B – 1).

The annual review should be used to re-evaluate the alert levels and, if necessary, modify them.

11.2 Equipment used for monitoring

11.2.1 Equipment used in monitoring should be calibrated at least annually by comparing with a traceable standard. A system should be in place to check all test certificates before signing the equipment back into use. Thermometers should be within 0.5°C (MHRA 2015), room pressure devices within 2Pa and HEPA filter pressure devices within 10% of the test device.

There is a requirement to monitor the storage temperature of microbial growth media, such as agar plates, aseptic manipulation kits and similar.

Pressure monitoring devices should be zeroed and calibrated to ensure warning and action levels are not breached.

11.2.2 Evidence should be available to demonstrate that environmental monitoring media are fit for purpose at the point of use.

The microbiological media used should be proven to be capable of supporting a broad spectrum of bacterial and fungal growth at the time of use.

This can be achieved by exposing a weekly positive control plate in an uncontrolled environment for sufficient time to provide a count of 5 or more after incubation.

11.2.3 Steps should be taken to ensure that surface sampling materials do not leave media residues; e.g. use of a sterile IMS wipe after sampling.

Microorganisms require water to reproduce and grow, and therefore leaving a surface wet after sampling with a moistened swab or contact plate could result in a proliferation of microbial contamination.

11.2.4 Plates should be labelled, wrapped in cling film or appropriately bagged as soon as possible after exposure and sent for incubation.

This is to ensure they do not become contaminated post exposure during transport to the laboratory and during incubation. The use of a plastic bag should be avoided if condensation becomes a problem as droplets of water falling on the agar surface during transportation could increase the count.

11.2.5 A negative control plate should be included on a weekly basis to check the plates are sterile and the post exposure handling, transport and incubation process does not introduce contamination.

11.2.6 Incubation should commence within seven days of exposure.

11.2.7 Liquid media such as Tryptone Soya Broth (TSB) used in aseptic validation kits should be assessed for fertility after use as described in Part B – 1.

11.3 Monitoring the aseptic preparation process

11.3.1 It is important that all staff, on commencing aseptic preparation, assure themselves that all equipment is functioning satisfactorily. Potential problems should be reported to senior staff.

A record should be made to demonstrate all checks have been completed as defined in local procedures.

11.3.2 When the unit is in use the critical zone of the controlled workspace should be monitored on a sessional basis. Settle plate exposure should seek to assess the worst case conditions – that is, capture microorganisms generated from the activity, for example, as close to the process in a EU GMP Grade A (EC 2015) environment as practical. For this to be successful, the way the plate is exposed is important and should form part of the standard operating procedure.

This may be achieved by the exposure of settle plates and undertaking a finger dab at the end of the work session.

Two settle plates should be used in two- or three- glove isolators or cabinets below 1.5 metres internal width and four plates should be exposed in four-glove isolators or cabinets 1.5 metres and above in width.

11.3.3 Passive air sampling using settle plates should be carried out for the full duration of the session. If sessions are longer than 4 hours, a second set of plates should be exposed.

11.3.4 When monitoring the clean room according to Table 11.1, one plate should be exposed in every aseptic preparation room and an additional plate per $12m^2$ floor area. Each room and each isolator transfer hatch should be monitored weekly.

Care should be taken in input hatches not to wet the agar with alcohol spray as it will affect the performance of the agar, inhibit growth and therefore could mask a problem. Care should also be taken to ensure maximum exposure of the agar by careful placement of the lid of the settle plate (See Part B –1).

11.3.5 Process validation using broth to simulate the aseptic procedure should be performed initially (three times is normal) and subsequently, at least on a 6 monthly basis. New processes or changes to existing processes, including the scale of activity, should be assessed to ensure previous validations remain valid (MHRA 2015).

A programme using different operators should be prepared. Process validation can form part of the periodic review of aseptic technique to supplement information from operator manipulation kits.

Comment: There is limited value in performing continuous particle monitoring for a manual closed process (MHRA 2015).

Automated processes require urgent intervention if the operation goes wrong and a continuous particle system can provide an alert for staff to check and, if necessary, stop the process. Manual operations such as opening syringe or needle packets, using low linting wipes or spraying disinfectant will generate particles sufficient to momentarily create a localised environment outside EU GMP Grade A (EC 2015). Quarterly occupied testing will allow an assessment of the particle generation inherent in the process as described in 11.6 for each workstation (MHRA 2015). The report should be risk assessed with reference to the aseptic procedures.

11.4 Environmental monitoring results

11.4.1 Alert limits for rooms should be established during commissioning. (Normally at least five sets of results should be obtained for each plate position.) The ideal methodology is to take the mean + 2 x standard deviation (95% value) or half the action limit, whichever is the smaller. Trending should be carried out to ensure the room remains in control. The alert limits should be reassessed during an annual review.

11.4.2 For pharmaceutical applications, the major criterion on which the aseptic facilities are assessed should be the risk of microbiological contamination of the product. Guideline action limits for microbiological data are given in Table 11.3. These limits are based on EU GMP (EC 2015) requirements.

Table 11.3
Environmental monitoring of controlled areas and clean air devices:
Action limits for microbiological tests in operation

GRADE	FINGER DABS CFU/HAND	SETTLE PLATES (90MM) CFU	CONTACT PLATE CFU/55MM DIAMETER	ACTIVE AIR SAMPLE CFU/M³
A (device)	< 1	< 1	< 1	< 1
B	Not applicable	5	5	10
C	Not applicable	50	25	100
D	Not applicable	100	50	200

Notes:
- Validated surface swabbing may be used as an alternative to contact plates. The same limits should be used for swabbing a 10 x 10cm area.
- Maximum exposure time for a settle plate is 4 hours.

11.4.3 If a plate exceeds the limits, the laboratory should assess the validity of the result and, if necessary, an out-of-specification review should be raised to determine whether the observation can be attributed to the test method or an artefact.

For example, if a finger dab plate is overgrown with colonies, it is unlikely to be associated with a finger but should nevertheless be investigated. A photograph of the plate may assist with the investigation.

11.4.4 Plates exposed in a gaseous biodecontamination isolator are expected to be clear after incubation. Any growth should be prioritised and identified to species level where possible.

Investigation by the aseptic unit staff should be carried out immediately. Guidance is given in Part B – 1.

11.4.5 Cabinets and isolators relying on liquid sanitisation of components will occasionally produce high counts due to the variability of bioburden and the efficiency of the process (Cockcroft 2001). If action levels are exceeded, growth should be identified to genus and preferably species level where possible.

Trending of results should be undertaken (see Part B – 1).

11.5   Testing the clean room environment and clean air devices

11.5.1 Equipment used in testing should be serviced and calibrated at least annually.

The test certificate is often presented as a set of results and the assessor should decide whether the equipment is fit for purpose before taking the equipment back into use.

11.5.2 In-use testing is important to provide assurance that procedures do not challenge aseptic manipulations with potentially viable particles. The assessment of airborne viable contamination should be carried out using an active air sampler (Part B – 1).

Use of an active air sampler will result in disturbance of air flow and could therefore impact on a product if being made at the time. It is therefore safer and often cost effective to carry out routine broth manipulation kits during quarterly environmental testing. Therefore, the choice of broth manipulation kit is important and all operators should be rostered in rotation to complete the kits. Sufficient kits to allow manipulations to occupy at least 20 minutes should be selected. Completing process validation manipulation kits has the greatest value (Part B – 2.1), however the Universal Operator Broth Transfer Validation Test (UOBTVT) includes a range of aseptic techniques and takes the required time to complete (Part B – 2.2).

A particle counter should be used to assess the total viable and non-viable particles.

Both the sampling devices should be positioned in the work area as close to the site of critical manipulations as possible without being knocked during operation. The active air sampler should be set to sample 1m³ of air and the particle counter should be set to repeatedly sample 10L of air. The tester needs to position themselves to allow the preparation process to be observed along with the particle count. If the particle counter display only monitors a single result it should be set to read 5μ. If the counter registers a 5μ count, the activity undertaken just before the count is recorded should be noted. The report should be analysed with reference to the SOPs for similar preparations. If particle counts are recorded whilst critical

QUALITY ASSURANCE OF ASEPTIC PREPARATION SERVICES:
STANDARDS HANDBOOK PART A

operations are being conducted, such as assembly of a syringe and needle or the puncture of a septum, the procedure may need to be changed to allow particles to disperse before the activity is conducted. This assessment is essential when turbulent flow has been identified e.g. using a smoke pencil.

11.5.3 The Filter integrity/Installation leak test (dispersed oil particulate (DOP) test) should be carried out on all supply HEPA filters.

The NHS specification for filters is given in table 11.5. DOP testing is often contracted out (see Part B – 3). The test forms the basis of acceptable viable and non-viable particle test results in the **'at rest'** state and therefore should be carried out by competent personnel. A protocol is available for guidance to ensure testing is carried out to NHS standards (PQAC 2010).

11.6 Environmental test results

11.6.1 Senior personnel concerned with aseptic preparation should have an understanding of clean room and clean air device technology, together with a thorough knowledge of all the particular design features in their department, e.g. ventilation systems, position and grade of HEPA filters, type of workstation, isolator design, etc. and the procedures carried out.

For pharmaceutical applications, the major criterion on which the aseptic facilities are assessed should be the risk of microbiological contamination of the product. However, because of the imprecision and variability of the microbiological test methods it is sometimes more practical to demonstrate environmental control using physical data. Guideline limits for physical and microbiological data in operation are given in Tables 11.3 and 11.4. These limits are based on EU GMP (EC 2015) requirements and BS EN ISO 14644 (BSI 1999b).

Note: For the annual retest using 'at rest' conditions, no preparation activity is carried out and the isolator or cabinet should be cleared of all items other than dedicated items such as cleaning materials. Therefore the test results should be used to determine whether there has been any deterioration since the previous test.

11.6.2 All areas associated with the aseptic preparation process should be assessed by the Accountable Pharmacist for compliance with the appropriate standards on commissioning, following maintenance procedures and routinely at an agreed frequency.

A written report of the test data indicating the significance of the results and recommended action should be brought to the attention of all relevant staff and full records kept on file for future reference.

'At rest' particle counts should be established during Operational Qualification and alert and action limits set.

For example, an isolator will typically not produce any particles > 0.5μ and therefore particle counts observed in the 'at rest' test could be a sign of fabric deterioration e.g. rust formation, particle build up due to inadequate cleaning or gaskets crumbling.

Table 11.4

Environmental monitoring of controlled areas and clean air devices:
Limits for physical tests

GRADE	PARTICLE COUNTS (MAXIMUM PARTICLES/M³)				AIR CHANGES (NUMBER PER HOUR)	PRESSURE DIFFERENTIAL PASCALS (PA) TO ADJACENT LOW CLASS AREA
	AT REST		IN OPERATION			
	0.5μm	5.0μm	0.5μm	5.0μm		
A (device)	3 520*	20*	3 520	20	Not applicable	Isolator >15 ****
B	3 520	29	352 000	2 900	> 30***	> 10
C	352 000	2 900	3 520 000	29 000	> 20	> 10
D	3 520 000	29 000	35 200 000	290 000**	> 20	>15

* It is recommended that tighter limits than EU GMP (EC 2015) 'at rest' are adopted for NHS aseptic units, for example based on commissioning data or calculated according to BS EN ISO 14644-1 (BSI 1999b). EU GMP Annex 1 (EC 2015) indicates that the 'in operation' and 'at rest' states should be defined for each room or suite of rooms.

** EU GMP (EC 2015) does not define the particle limits for 'in operation' for a EU GMP Grade D (EC 2015) room. It is recommended that the room is tested and BS EN ISO Class 9 (BSI 2015) is adopted.

*** The number of air changes per hour can be less than the values stated in table 11.4 provided it can be demonstrated that the room will return to the 'at rest' conditions within 20 minutes. (This is referred to as the recovery or 'clean up' rate). These figures are the usual minimum specification for new facilities, however under all conditions a minimum of 20 air changes per hour should be achieved.

**** Minimum recommendation for isolators used to manipulate cytotoxic drug substances (HSE and MHRA 2015).

It is important that the required clean up time of 20 minutes is achieved (EC 2015).

QUALITY ASSURANCE OF ASEPTIC PREPARATION SERVICES:
STANDARDS HANDBOOK PART A

Table 11.5
HEPA filter classification and testing for aseptic preparation

EU GMP GRADE (EC 2015) OF ENVIRONMENT	MINIMUM CLASSIFICATION OF FILTER (BSI 2009)	DOP TEST MINIMUM (PQAC 2010)
A and B	H14	≤0.001%
C and D	H13	≤0.01%

Note:
Any deviation from these limits should be fully documented and justified by the Accountable Pharmacist.

11.7 Sterility testing and/or end of session broth tests

11.7.1 A documented sterility test programme should be in place, which includes consideration of all process variables. The minimum expectation is one sterility test per operational work station per week. Variables such as product and operators should be cyclically covered on a rolling basis. This sterility testing frequency only applies where there is sufficient data to demonstrate that the areas are adequately controlled and therefore would not initially apply for new facilities where there is no history. Any sterility test failures should be identified to species (and preferably strain) level and thoroughly investigated.

11.7.2 The use of a suitably designed 'end of session media fill simulation' may be considered as an alternative to sterility testing of the finished product as part of an on-going monitoring programme.

End of session broth tests (EOS) can be developed (MHRA 2015) using TSB (Part B – I). The EOS test should be designed to incorporate similar components and processes used in the preparation of aseptic products. Broth can be used to fill items used in a preparation, however, residues of product should not impede the ability of the medium to support microorganism growth. This does not completely remove the requirement to carry out sterility tests, but could justify reducing the frequency to monthly.

It is not recommended that an EOS kit is used for radiopharmaceutical preparation using a ^{99m}Tc generator as it is important to assure the sterility of the generator throughout its use (Society of Nuclear Medicine 2006) and this cannot be achieved through use of an EOS.

11.7.3 If an end of session broth test fails, an investigation should be undertaken. If there is no satisfactory explanation, the result should be treated as operator broth transfer validation test failure (see Chapter 9: Personnel, training and competency assessment) and corrective and/or preventative action (CAPA) undertaken.

11.8 Monitoring of finished products

11.8.1 There should be a planned programme of physical, chemical and microbiological analysis of the finished product, as appropriate.

11.8.2 Samples may be obtained from:

- unused products
- additional specially-prepared samples
- an in-process sample taken at the end of the compounding procedure before the final seals are in place and before removal from the critical zone.

11.8.3 Sampling of the final container after completion of preparation and prior to issue may be a threat to product integrity and is therefore not recommended.

11.8.4 The testing laboratory should be fully conversant with the technical background and requirements in aseptic preparation, together with the validated methodology for analysing the products and samples. The Accountable Pharmacist should ensure that the testing laboratory has a comprehensive knowledge of pharmaceutical microbiology.

11.8.5 A technical agreement should be in place with the providers of any external testing services and this should be monitored. (An example of a technical agreement is given in Part B – 3).

11.9 Sink and drain monitoring

All sinks, wash-stations and drains associated with the clean room suite, as well as social hand washing sinks, should be monitored.

Hot and cold tap water supplies should be tested on commissioning and monitored on a quarterly basis by total viable count (TVC) to ensure the water is not heavily contaminated (see Part B – 1). A limit of 100cfu/ml has historically been adopted for potable water. Drains should be similarly monitored (WHO 2003).

If the limit is exceeded, identification of the genus of the organisms present is advised.

Organisms that form biofilms (such as pseudomonads) and other Gram negative organisms should trigger treatment. The water system should be flushed for a minimum of 2 minutes and the water retested. If the supply continues to fail the TVC due to pseudomonads or other Gram negative organisms, the estates department should be asked to look at the supply as described in HTM 04 01 (DH 2006).

Drains: if the limit is exceeded, then the drains should be flushed with water for a minimum of 2 minutes and subjected to either the designated heated trap exposure or suitable chemical disinfection and retested.

Note: For water sampling from sinks and drains conditions see Part B – 1, BSI 1999a.

11.10 Planned preventative maintenance

It is important not to confuse PPM with testing. The aim of PPM is to prevent a process from failing due to a defective piece of equipment. There should be a PPM plan in place for all critical pieces of equipment.

11.10.1 A technical agreement should be in place for PPM of all critical pieces of equipment detailing frequency, permits to work, responsibilities, expected tasks and actions and reporting mechanism (see Part B – 3).

For isolators, the PPM schedule should concentrate on the integrity of the carcass by paying particular attention to changing seals and gaskets, and tightening bolts and screws. Indicator light operation, door timer checks and gauge calibration are often overlooked. The leak test should be recorded before and after PPM activity and the results used to determine whether the unit is deteriorating between visits.

An assessment of the performance of the fans for all cabinets and air handling systems will provide an early warning if a fan requires replacing and prevent a failure of the equipment.

11.10.2 All reports should be assessed by the Accountable Pharmacist against the technical agreement to ensure all work has been carried out and the outcome is satisfactory. If not, appropriate action should be taken to remedy any deficiencies.

References

British Standards Institute (BSI) (1999a). *BS EN ISO 6222:1999. Water quality - Enumeration of culturable micro organisms - Colony count by inoculation in a nutrient agar culture medium.* London: BSI

British Standards Institute (BSI) (1999b). *BS EN ISO 14644-1:1999. Clean Rooms and Associated Controlled Environments. Part 1: Classification of Air Cleanliness.* London: BSI.

British Standards Institute (BSI) (2000). *BS EN 12469:2000. Biotechnology-Performance Criteria for Microbiological Safety Cabinets.* Milton Keynes: BSI.

British Standards Institute (BSI) (2009). *BS EN 1822-1:2009. High Efficiency Air Filters (HEPA and ULPA) Classifications, Performance Testing and Marking.* Milton Keynes: BSI.

British Standards Institute (BSI) (2015). *BS EN ISO 14644-1:2015. Clean Rooms and Associated Controlled Environments. Classification of Air Cleanliness by Particle Concentration.* London: BSI.

Cockcroft MG et al (2001). Validation of liquid disinfection techniques for transfer of components into hospital pharmacy clean rooms. *Hospital Pharmacy* 8: 226-232.

Department of Health (DH) (2006). Health Technical Memorandum HTM 04-01. *The control of Legionella, hygiene, 'safe' hot water, cold water and drinking water systems.* Norwich: The Stationery Office.

European Commission (2015). *The rules governing medicinal products in the European Community. Vol IV. Good Manufacturing Practice for medicinal products.* Available at: **http://ec.europa.eu/health/documents/eudralex/vol-4/index_en.htm** (accessed 26 February 2016).

Farwell J (1995). *Aseptic Dispensing for NHS Patients.* (The Farwell Report). London: Department of Health.

Health and Safety Executive (HSE) and Medicines and Healthcare products Regulatory Agency (MHRA) (2015). *Handling cytotoxic drugs in isolators in NHS pharmacies.* Sudbury: Health and Safety Executive.

Hiom SJ et al (2004). Development and validation of a method to assess alcohol transfer disinfection procedures. *Pharm J* 272: 611.

Medicines and Healthcare products Regulatory Agency (MHRA) (2015). *Questions and Answers for Specials Manufacturers.* London: MHRA. Available at: **www.gov.uk/government/publications/guidance-for-specials-manufacturers** (accessed 19 February 2016).

Midcalf B et al (2004). *Pharmaceutical Isolators.* London: Pharmaceutical Press.

Needle R, Sizer T eds (1998). *The CIVAS Handbook.* London: Pharmaceutical Press.

NHS Pharmaceutical Quality Assurance Committee (PQAC) (2010). *DOP testing of HEPA filters.*

Parenteral Drug Association (PDA) (1980). *Validation of Aseptic Filling for Solution Drug Products: Technical Monograph No 2.* Maryland: Parenteral Drug Association.

Pharmaceutical and Healthcare Sciences Society (PHSS) (2002). *Environmental Contamination Control Practice: Technical Monograph No 2.* Swindon: Pharmaceutical and Healthcare Sciences Society.

Pharmaceutical Inspection Co-operation Scheme (PIC/S) (2007). *Isolators used for aseptic processing and sterility testing.* PI 014-3. Geneva: PIC/S.

Society of Nuclear Medicine (2006). Mallinckrodt Issues ^{99m}Tc Generator Recall (news). *The Journal of Nuclear Medicine* 47(1): p26N. Available at: **http://jnm.snmjournals.org/content/47/1.toc** (accessed 18 February 2016).

UK Radiopharmacy Group (UKRG) and NHS Pharmaceutical Quality Assurance Committee (PQAC) (2012). *Quality Assurance of Radiopharmaceuticals.* Available at: **www.bnms.org.uk/images/stories/UKRG/UKRG_QA_Apr-12.pdf** (accessed 26 February 2016).

World Health Organisation (WHO) (2003). Ed Bartram J et al. *Heterotrophic plate counts and drinking-water safety: The significance of HPCs for water quality and the human health.* London: IWA Publishing.

CHAPTER 12 CLEANING, SANITISATION AND BIODECONTAMINATION

Clean air devices, in combination with the design, structure and use of clean rooms, are intended to provide a clean environment in which to prepare sterile medicines. Therefore the sanitisation of clean areas is particularly important (EC 2015). There are a number of ways to reduce contamination, including cleaning, sanitisation, disinfection and biodecontamination.

It is important to remember that surfaces in clean rooms, and clean air devices, together with the surfaces of starting materials, components and consumables, can become contaminated with microorganisms over time, even if the area is not occupied.

These surfaces of starting materials, components and consumables present a considerable risk because of the potential to transfer the contamination into the critical zone.

Therefore, the appropriate use of cleaning and disinfecting agents (that is, sanitisation) are important parts of the contamination control programme.

12.1 General principles

12.1.1 All sanitisation processes should be undertaken regularly in accordance with a written programme and subject to standard operating procedures.

12.1.2 All cleaning and disinfecting agents employed in the clean room facility should be subject to a formal, documented assessment and approval process.

12.1.3 Where disinfectants are used, more than one type should be employed to reduce the risk of the development of resistance in microorganisms.

Environmental monitoring data should be regularly reviewed to highlight trends that might suggest the presence of resistant organisms or spores (see Chapter 11: Monitoring).

12.1.4 Cleaning and disinfecting agents should be free from viable microorganisms. Those used in Grade A and B areas should be sterile prior to use (EC 2015).

It is advisable that all controlled areas including EU GMP Grades C and D (EC 2015) should use sterile water as a diluent when needed.

12.1.5 Wherever possible, sterile ready-to-use agents should be used. If not, in-use dilutions should be freshly prepared for each cleaning session. Samples from freshly-prepared dilutions should be monitored for microbiological contamination at least once every six months.

12.1.6 Wet or damp cleaning with effective detergents should be the method of choice. (Disinfectants only work when wet.) Dry dusting alone is not recommended but dedicated vacuum cleaners with the appropriate control (that is, HEPA filtered) may be used to remove any dust and debris.

12.1.7 The following factors should be considered when choosing a sanitisation process:

- efficacy of the sanitisation agent to achieve sufficient coverage to achieve microbial kill
- contact time, evaporation rate, air flow over the surface and air change rate
- organic and inorganic load present in the unit, including drug residues
- type and level of microbial contamination (bioburden)
- physical nature of the object (e.g. crevices, folds, hinges, and lumens)
- presence of biofilms
- other factors such as relative humidity involved in biodecontamination
- other factors such as health and safety and presentation etc.

12.1.8 The use of sanitisation agents should be controlled according to a documented procedure/policy and this should include:

- a statement of the in-use shelf life, which should be justified and documented. Information from manufacturers may be acceptable, subject to critical appraisal.
- an indication on any container of sanitisation agent as to the date of opening. (Processes in place should ensure that these are not used beyond the specified in-use shelf life.)
- a requirement that storage of in-house diluted sanitisation agents is not permitted. These should be prepared in previously cleaned containers with sterile water and used immediately.
- steps to limit operator variability in-use e.g. a defined training programme, detailed procedures for preparation and application etc.

- for purchased items, an assurance from the manufacturer regarding the quality and effectiveness of the supplied item and confirmation that the product is sterile if specified.
- for items sterilised by irradiation, evidence that this process has been completed satisfactorily (e.g. proof of activity/absence of degradation).
- during use, processes to ensure that the external surfaces of any container of the sanitisation agent itself are sanitised such that it does not present a risk of contamination during use.

12.1.9 Sterile water, and where appropriate, sterile non-foaming detergents, should be used periodically to ensure the removal of residues, e.g. of medicines and disinfectants, biofilms, dirt and grease.

12.1.10 Logs should be kept of the areas cleaned indicating the agents used. These should be checked for compliance before use of the facility and reviewed periodically.

12.1.11 All staff performing any cleaning duties should have received documented training, including the relevant elements of EU GMP (EC 2015) and specific information relating to the agents and methods employed. Cleaners should be assessed to be competent before being allowed to work unsupervised.

12.1.12 There should be continuity of cleaning staff with the provision of adequate suitably trained cover. Any contract cleaners should be subject to a technical (quality) agreement which is closely monitored (see Part B – 3).

12.1.13 The effectiveness of cleaning should be routinely demonstrated by review of the surface monitoring programme employed; both microbiological and chemical (see Chapter 11: Monitoring).

12.1.14 Surface monitoring results should be trended. If these show an increase in microbiological contamination, change in microbial flora, or the presence of objectionable organisms, the prompt use of additional cleaning and/or the use of alternative disinfectants should be considered.

12.1.15 Surface monitoring for residues (in particular, hazardous materials such as cytotoxic agents) should be routinely undertaken (minimum annually) and trending carried out. The sites chosen for residue monitoring should reflect the perceived highest risk areas.

Cleaning regimens should be demonstrated to effectively remove chemical contamination. If residues persist, prompt use of additional cleaning and/or the use of alternative products should be considered. The chemistry and solubility of the residues should be considered to ensure effective removal.

12.2 Cleaning the facility

The correct level of cleanliness should be achieved by a well-designed facility which is maintained in a clean and dry status (see Chapter 7: Facilities and equipment).

Note: Fumigation of clean areas may be useful for reducing microbiological contamination in inaccessible places or in the situation of gross contamination. Such processes, if used, should be validated and documented.

12.2.1 Controlled areas should be regularly cleaned according to a written, approved procedure and, when necessary, disinfected using validated and approved agents. Cleaning of outer areas of the facility is equally important to minimise the entry of contamination into the controlled areas.

Table 12.1
Minimum recommended cleaning frequencies

	CEILING	WALLS	FLOORS	HANDLES AND SWITCHES	BENCHES AND TROLLEYS (UNDERSIDES)	MISCELLANEOUS EQUIPMENT, E.G. EXTERNAL SURFACES OF CLEAN AIR DEVICES, FRIDGES ETC.
Grade B	3M	M	D	D	D (3M)	W
Grade C	6M	3M	D	D	D (3M)	W
Grade D	A	3M	W	D	D (3M)	M
Unclassified e.g Outer support areas		A	W	W	W	M
Stores			W	W	W	M
Sinks and hand wash stations	As a minimum, sinks and hand wash-stations should be cleaned daily including taps and other fitments. Drains and traps should be disinfected regularly (minimum weekly). Taps should be flushed for 2 minutes before use on a daily basis (DH 2012).					

A - annually, M - monthly, W - weekly, D - daily

Note:
The above frequencies are based on regular daily usage of the environment concerned. Where rooms or equipment are used intermittently, cleaning and monitoring regimens may need to be amended following an appropriate and documented risk assessment.

12.2.2 Dedicated clean room cleaning equipment should be used appropriate to the grade of room, e.g. sterile in EU GMP Grade B (EC 2015).

12.2.3 Clean room cleaning equipment should be stored separately from all other cleaning materials and securely so that it is not used in the incorrect areas, and to minimise microbiological contamination.

12.2.4 The facility should be cleaned in a defined order.

This normally means that the cleaning process starts in the cleanest grade area and progresses outwards to the areas with the lowest grade of cleanliness. It is usual to begin at high level and finish at low level and to work from the point furthest from the door to the point nearest the door.

Best practice is to apply cleaning agents with separate, overlapping stroke techniques in defined directions.

12.2.5 For EU GMP Grade B (EC 2015) areas mopheads should be sterile, low-linting, disposable and intended for single use only, or they may be resterilised after each cleaning session. This sterilisation process should be validated and subject to regular review.

12.2.6 All methods of application, including preloaded mops, should deliver enough of the product to achieve effective cleaning and/or disinfection for the full period of contact to the defined area.

Pooling of excess amounts of cleaning or disinfecting agents should be avoided. Ideally surfaces should become dry within 1 hour of application. Conversely, sufficient product should remain to achieve the required efficacy throughout the recommended contact time i.e. disinfectants should not be spread too thinly.

12.2.7 Adhesive flooring designed to remove soiling from footwear and the wheels of equipment should be incorporated into cleaning schedules.

Those contamination control floor coverings intended for reuse should be cleaned and regenerated regularly with manufacturer's approved agents. When using tacky mats, the normal minimum expectation is that each foot should impact with the mat twice. Wheeled vehicles should travel in straight lines and not turn on the surface of the mat as this can cause permanent damage.

Those intended for removal should be replaced as soon as soiling is seen to be unacceptable. Such removal or cleaning should be performed to minimise the liberation of particles. Every effort should be made to remove any adhesive residues resulting from placement of these mats.

12.3 Clean air devices

12.3.1 Clean air devices should be cleaned and disinfected before and after each working session with approved sterile agents (typically 70% alcohol).

12.3.2 Internal work surfaces of clean air devices should have a periodic sporicidal clean (minimum monthly, or where monitoring results dictate, or following an incident, e.g. a spillage, sleeve replacement etc.).

All traces of sporicide should be removed after an appropriate contact time, e.g. with 70% sterile alcohol wipes.

For gaseous biodecontamination isolators, a clean of the internal surfaces with a non-ionic sterile detergent should be carried out before vapourised hydrogen peroxide (VHP) gassing (**Note:** IMS wipes can cause interference with hydrogen peroxide sensors and are therefore not recommended).

12.3.3 Periodically all clean room surfaces, particularly the external surfaces of clean air devices, should be cleaned with an agent that will remove chemical residues (at a minimum quarterly frequency).

These might include sterile agents, such as neutral detergent, water, or acidified water and a weak alkali wash, depending on the nature of the materials handled.

12.3.4 All surfaces, both internal and external, should be cleaned in accordance with a written schedule with attention given to difficult-to-access nooks and crannies. Installed equipment should follow a similar regime.

12.4 Gaseous biodecontamination

12.4.1 The ability to decontaminate isolators with a sporicidal gaseous agent should be considered at the time of purchase of a new isolator.

Gaseous agents such as VHP or ionised hydrogen peroxide (IHP) have good profiles as bactericides, and fungicides and importantly as sporicides. They can be utilised for the decontamination of the internal surfaces of an isolator as well as for the transfer disinfection process.

The use of spray and wipe techniques remain acceptable as a method of transfer disinfection. However, if a new unit or isolator is required, the use of gassing technology should be taken into consideration and a risk assessment performed (MHRA 2015).

12.4.2 Biodecontamination should be performed in a controlled manner, that is, the process should be reproducible, with a defined microbiological kill profile, load profile and an independent processing record. The cycle should be automatic, recorded on a printout, and reviewed (including any alarms) to confirm acceptability.

12.4.3 Physical cleaning of isolators employing biodecontamination is required in addition to the decontamination process, however.

12.5 Transfer disinfection processes

Surface disinfection of components prior to the transfer is vital in preventing the ingress of contamination into critical areas.

The design of the transfer disinfection process is of utmost importance. As an alternative to liquid sanitisation, the use of irradiated triple-wrapped products should be considered as it can improve the sterility assurance of the process. The use of multi-packs or user specific preparation kits can be beneficial.

Note: Further guidance and advice is available (PQAC 2015).

12.5.1 The process should have a written standard operating procedure and should be validated.

12.5.2 Sterile agents should be used in EU GMP Grade A and B (EC 2015) zones and during the last sanitisation stages of the transfer disinfection process (MHRA 2015).

Best practice is that sterile agents are used throughout the transfer disinfection process to reduce the risk of selecting the incorrect agent.

Note: Although 70% alcohol solutions are widely used, these are not sporicidal (Cockcroft et al 2001). Spores should be removed both by a physical wiping stage in the surface sanitisation procedure and by the application of a sporicidal agent such as hydrogen peroxide or chlorine-based agents (MHRA 2015).

12.5.3 The contact time should be clearly stated, validated and maintained in practice. The minimum period for contact with a disinfectant in the transfer process is 2 minutes. Evidence should be available to substantiate the effectiveness of this contact time.

It is assumed that starting materials and components used for aseptic preparation such as needles, luer connections etc. are transferred into a support room, stored, with subsequent transfer through airlocks into the clean room and then into a clean air device.

12.5.4 The storage of paper and cardboard in the support room should also be minimised, whilst at the same time ensuring that the product is protected, e.g. from light, and secure and key information, e.g. the Summary of Product Characteristics (SmPC), is still available to allow correct use of the product.

12.5.5 Before transfer to the clean room, a sanitisation step using a wipe and spray technique including a sporicidal agent designed to inactivate bacterial and fungal spores should be carried out. (Step 1).

12.5.6 Before transfer to the working zone a second sanitisation step using a spray and wipe technique including a disinfectant should be carried out. (Step 2).

12.5.7 The minimum expectation is therefore two discrete decontamination steps, with a spray and wipe performed at both steps and the first decontamination step should use a sporicidal agent.

Spraying should take place as the product is transferred into the transfer hatch. This activity should not be remote from the hatch.

12.5.8 The only exemption from using a sporicidal agent in step 1, at the current time, is for radiopharmaceuticals and biologically-derived medicines, but only where evidence is available that the product performance may be affected by sporicidal residues (MHRA 2015). Evidence for radiopharmaceuticals is available (Dadda et al 2014, Fisher et al 1977, Murray et al 1986, Stringer et al 1997, Verbruggen et al 1985). Justification may be possible in other circumstances, however documentation to support the approach taken should be available. In these situations, a four-stage disinfection process with alcohol is required. Serious consideration should also be given to other methods of transfer to minimise the risk of bacterial and fungal spores entering the critical zone, e.g. use of irradiated double- and triple-wrapped components.

12.5.9 During sanitisation, particular attention should be paid to the rubber septa of vials and break lines of ampoules, which should be subjected to all stages of the sanitisation treatment. Over-seals (e.g. flip-off caps) should therefore be removed at the first sanitisation stage.

It is important to ensure that the disinfectant gets into all difficult to access areas such as under the crimp seal of vials.

12.5.10 An effective contact time for the sanitising agent should be used. Third party supplier data may be used, provided that this is reviewed to demonstrate its relevance to the intended use. Where contact time differs from the manufacturer's recommendations, this should be supported by scientifically valid microbiological studies.

Consideration should also be given to the air classification of the support room and a risk assessment should be performed where this room is unclassified to consider if any additional controls are required.

12.5.11 The following factors should be considered in development of a surface sanitisation strategy:

- The bioburden challenge presented by the type of item being sanitised, i.e. number of surfaces and ease of cleaning
- The minimum residence period post sanitisation (2 minutes is usually applied as a guidance value for a disinfectant effect. Longer times may be required for a sporicidal effect)
- Periodic verification of sanitisation effectiveness. (This should be carried out with frequency based on a risk assessment)
- Any extended storage time for sanitised components. (This is considered to be a risk factor, and subsequent sanitisation steps prior to use should address this risk)
- Minimising the exposure time of items supplied as sterile prior to entering the EU GMP Grade A (EC 2015) critical zone to reduce the risk of contamination
- The requirement for any folds on the surface of sealed packages to be sanitised
- The effective shelf life of products in use.

12.5.12 Consideration should also be given to other methods (e.g. irradiated double- and triple-wrapped components) to minimise the transfer of bacterial and fungal spores.

12.6 Additional requirements concerning transfer disinfection processes

12.6.1 Clothing requirements: As a minimum requirement, gloves should be worn for all transfer disinfection processes. These should be sterile or disinfected before use.

Best practice is that a non-shedding protective coat or suit, face mask, clean room shoes and suitable headwear are worn to protect the product and operator during transfer disinfection processes (see Chapter 7: Facilities and equipment).

12.6.2 Operator technique: It is essential that a high degree of diligence and attention to detail is applied. The standard operating procedure should define the process and be followed. Routine supervision of this activity is required.

12.6.3 Wiping technique: Impregnated wipes should be used in preference to dry wipes (the latter being wetted in situ).

Evidence indicates that dry wipes are rarely wetted enough to readily release sufficient liquid onto the surface. In addition, the undulating and micro-structures of surfaces being disinfected do not facilitate the effective delivery of disinfectant by the wipe process (Panousi et al 2009).

12.6.4 Wipes used should be low linting and be sterile when used at the last step of transfer for aseptic products.

Although natural fibre wipes may potentially shed more particulates, they have the advantage of increased wickability over most synthetic materials, holding more liquid and therefore releasing more disinfectant to kill surface-borne organisms. They also entrap particles and absorb residues more readily.

The roles and uses of the wipes are:

- *To physically remove the bioburden from the surface*
- *To ensure the presence of sufficient disinfectant for long enough to kill vegetative and, where needed, spore-forming organisms*
- *To facilitate the destruction and removal of contaminants by the application of pressure against microbial cell walls during the wiping process.*

12.6.5 For non-sporicidal wipes, a fresh surface of each wipe is required to prevent the transfer of dirt and bioburden from the wipe to other surfaces.

This can be achieved by systematically folding the wipe. Care should be taken to ensure that surfaces are not reused.

12.6.6 Wiping technique should follow defined wipe patterns, with additional care taken for cleaning in folds, the rubber septa of vials, and the break lines of ampoules.

12.6.7 The initial bioburden of container surfaces should be well-controlled and regularly monitored (minimum annually). Starting materials, components and consumables should be stored to minimise bioburden.

12.6.8 Health and safety aspects should be considered for relevant disinfecting and biodecontamination agents, in particular sporicidal agents, and also for dealing with spillages of chemicals and products, e.g. cytotoxics.

This may be demonstrated by contemporary COSHH (The Control of Substances Hazardous to Health Regulations 2002) records and risk assessments.

12.7 Tray cleaning

12.7.1 In addition to routine spraying and wiping with liquid disinfectant, trays used for the transfer of components into clean rooms and clean air devices should be designed to be easily cleanable. They should be washed and decontaminated periodically. The frequency should be justified and defined by local practice and needs.

12.7.2 Tray cleaning should not take place in the clean or controlled support area. Tray cleaning should be in a suitable location.

Sinks, hand wash-stations and basins used for hand washing should be avoided for health and safety reasons (e.g. the exposure to cytotoxics).

12.7.3 Following washing, trays should be dried, disinfected, and returned into the aseptic suite. Trays should not be left to 'drain'.

12.7.4 Tray cleaning should be periodically validated. Annual revalidation is suggested.

12.8 Hand washing

Hand contamination, whether gloved or ungloved, also poses a considerable risk to the clean environment, as this is probably the greatest potential for transferring microbial contamination.

12.8.1 The use of appropriate hand hygiene techniques, hand disinfectants and gloving technique is a vital part of good contamination control.

12.8.2 The choice of disinfectant for hand sanitisation, as well as the techniques utilised, should be effective against the types of microorganisms likely to be present.

Note: Ordinary hand wash agents (e.g. soap) are not suitable on their own for use in the clean room environment. Antimicrobial agents such as chlorhexidine and iodophors are recommended.

12.8.3 Hand washing effectiveness should be assessed and documented.

12.8.4 Hand washing facilities should be located outside of, and adjacent to, the clean room suite. In a new unit, hand washing facilities should be located next to the main entrance of the clean room suite.

In older facilities, the use of hand basins within the toilet facilities may be permitted providing they are cleaned daily. In addition, hands cleaned in such hand basins should be further treated by the application of an alcoholic hand gel prior to entry to the clean room suite.

12.8.5 Hand washing facilities and the water supplied to them should be regularly monitored for compliance with appropriate limits, e.g. the EU limits for potable water are 100cfu/ml at 25°C and 10cfu/ml at 35°C (see Chapter 11: Monitoring). Taps should be flushed each day that the unit is in use (see Table 12.1).

12.9 Cleaning validation

12.9.1 Periodic verification of sanitisation effectiveness should be carried out, with frequency based on risk assessment. This applies to general cleaning of the environment and specifically to transfer disinfection.

The following are suggested minimum frequencies:

Table 12.2
Suggested minimum sampling frequencies for cleaning validation

	MICROBIOLOGY	CHEMICAL
Hand wash	Annual	Not applicable
Transfer disinfection	6 Monthly	Not applicable
Critical zone	6 Monthly	Annual
Room cleaning	Annual	Annual

Notes:
Cleaning validation should consider the level of contamination before and after cleaning.
Chemical decontamination should consider product residues, and possibly, disinfectant residues.
Tray cleaning should be periodically validated. Annual revalidation is suggested.

12.9.2 Limits should be established locally, and be based upon both microbiological and chemical residue analysis.

QUALITY ASSURANCE OF ASEPTIC PREPARATION SERVICES:
STANDARDS HANDBOOK PART A

References

Cockcroft MG et al (2001). Validation of liquid disinfection techniques for transfer of components into hospital pharmacy clean rooms. *Hospital Pharmacy* 8: 226-232.

Dadda, A et al (2014). Determination of Sn2+ in lyophilized radiopharmaceuticals by voltammetry, using hydrochloric acid as electrolyte. *J Braz Chem Soc* 25(9): 1621-1629. Available at: ***http://jbcs.sbq.org.br/imagebank/pdf/v25n9a11.pdf*** (accessed 03 March 2016).

Department of Health (2012). *Health Technical Memorandum 04-01 – Addendum: Pseudomonas aeruoginosa – advice for augmented care units.*

European Commission (2015). *The rules governing medicinal products in the European Community. Vol IV. Good Manufacturing Practice for medicinal products.* Available at: ***http://ec.europa.eu/health/documents/eudralex/vol-4/index_en.htm*** (accessed 26 February 2016).

Fisher SM, et al (1977). Unbinding of ^{99m}Tc by Iodinated Antiseptics. *The Journal of Nuclear Medicine* 18:1139-1140. Available at: ***http://jnm.snmjournals.org/content/18/11/1139.2.citation*** (accessed 15 April 2016).

Medicines and Healthcare products Regulatory Agency (MHRA) (2015). *Questions and Answers for Specials Manufacturers.* London: MHRA. Available at: ***www.gov.uk/government/publications/guidance-for-specials-manufacturers*** (accessed 19 February 2016).

Murray T et al (1986). Formation of Labelled Colloid in ^{99m}Tc-DMSA due to the Presence of Bactericidal Fluid *Nuclear Med Commun* 7: 505-510.

NHS Pharmaceutical Quality Assurance Committee (PQAC) (2015). *Guidance for Aseptic Transfer Processes in the NHS: Addressing Sporicidal Issues.* NHS PhQAC Advice Notice: Sporicides in the Aseptic Transfer Process 2015.

Panousi MN et al (2009). Evaluation of alcohol wipes used during aseptic manufacturing. *Lett Appl Microbiol* 48(5): 648-51. Abstract. Available at: ***www.ncbi.nlm.nih.gov/pubmed/19228287*** (accessed 04 March 2016).

Stringer RE et al (1997). MAG3 failure is due to inadvertent oxidant contamination. *Nuclear Medicine Communications.* 18: 294.

The Control of Substances Hazardous to Health Regulations (COSHH) 2002. SI 2002 No. 2677. London: The Stationery Office ***www.legislation.gov.uk/uksi/2002/2677/pdfs/uksi_20022677_en.pdf*** (accessed 04 February 2016).

Verbruggen A, et al. (1985). Interaction between some Disinfectants and ^{99m}Tc Radiopharmaceuticals Progress in Radiopharmacology. In: *Developments in Nuclear Medicine.* Dordrecht: Martinus Nijhoff Publishers. 239-250.

QUALITY ASSURANCE OF ASEPTIC PREPARATION SERVICES:
STANDARDS HANDBOOK PART A

CHAPTER 13 STARTING MATERIALS, COMPONENTS AND CONSUMABLES

There need to be robust systems in place to control the quality of starting materials, components and consumables used in the preparation of medicines. Lack of control can have a direct impact on overall product quality.

Management of change in the supply of materials should be carefully controlled and monitored to ensure no additional risks are introduced.

13.1 Starting materials

This term applies to all materials used in the preparation of a medicinal product, excluding components or consumables but including any re-worked products (see below). These materials may also be termed ingredients.

13.1.1 Starting materials should be sterile products and should preferably have a Marketing Authorisation. Unlicensed starting materials should not be used where there is a licensed equivalent available. (MHRA 2014).

13.1.2 Where unlicensed starting materials are used, it is incumbent on the Accountable Pharmacist to ensure that the product is of the appropriate quality by means of specifications, certificates of analysis or conformity, quality control tests or a combination of these. This assessment should be documented and be in accordance with the organisation's unlicensed medicines policy.

13.1.3 Unlicensed starting materials should always be obtained from a manufacturer with an appropriate manufacturer's licence. Supply of medicines licensed in countries outside of the UK, often via an importer, may be acceptable but should be in accordance with the unlicensed medicines policy.

13.1.4 For licensed starting materials, systems for receipt should also include verification that the Summary of Product Characteristics or technical information supplied has not changed since the previous receipt. Where changes are noted, there should be an impact assessment conducted and if the change requires a modification then change management procedures should be invoked.

13.1.5 For unpreserved starting materials, the in-use shelf life should be restricted to one aseptic work session (not exceeding 4 hours) during which the material remains in the critical zone (PQAC 2014).

13.1.6 Similar starting materials for each product should be sourced from the same manufacturer i.e. no mixed strengths of the same material from different manufacturers.

The formulation from one manufacturer may differ from that of another and has the risk of incompatibility or effect on shelf life (see Chapter 6: Formulation, stability and shelf life).

13.1.7 Non-sterile starting materials should never be used.

13.1.8 Any material that is re-worked should be treated as a new starting material. The re-working of a product transforms it into a starting material. Its suitability for use should be assessed as for any other starting material.

13.1.9 Ampoules should only ever be used for a single withdrawal immediately after opening and then discarded under the description of a closed procedure (PQAC 2014).

13.1.10 The sharing of vials of starting materials between patients is an acceptable process provided that it is carried out on a campaign basis and is subject to robust risk assessment (PQAC 2014).

A campaign basis means that two or more doses may be drawn up from the same vial or the same pool of vials as long as these doses are made sequentially, that no other products are present in the work zone throughout the process, and that the vials stay within the Grade A work zone throughout the process.

13.1.11 Vial sharing for single use vials outside of pharmacy aseptic units is unacceptable (PQAC 2014).

13.2 Components and other consumables

Critical components include:

- Syringes and caps used as final containers
- Connecting sets used for compounding purposes.

Other components include:

- Reconstitution devices
- Venting devices
- Syringes and needles not used as final container
- Parts of filling systems in direct contact with the product.

Consumables include:

- Alcohol sprays
- Wipes (including cleaning tool covers)
- Other cleaning agents and materials
- Sharps bins
- Trays.

13.2.1 Components should be purchased pre-sterilised from the manufacturer. The product should be either a CE marked medical device or have a documented form of approval. It should be packaged in such a way that it can be passed into the aseptic environment without increasing the risk of product or environmental contamination.

13.2.2 Any filters used should be pre-assembled by the manufacturer, CE marked and guaranteed sterile.

13.2.3 There should be a record of batch numbers on the worksheet for critical components (see Chapter 8: Pharmaceutical Quality System).

13.2.4 Batch traceability for other components should be available to enable the audit trail in the event of a recall. A log may be used for this purpose.

13.2.5 Local sterilisation of non-sterile consumables and equipment is acceptable provided that sterility is assured. Such sterilisation processes should be validated, appropriately monitored and meet all current standards. (DH 2013, BSI 2012). Assurance should be given that there is no risk of cross contamination from surgical instruments or other types of non-pharmaceutical activity. An audit trail should be available. A Technical Agreement is required with some evidence of periodic audit of the sterilising site. (See Part B – 3).

13.2.6 Filling systems should not be modified.

13.2.7 Sterile components should be stored so as to minimise any increase in the bioburden on the surface of the primary and secondary packaging. All items should be appropriately stored to prevent damage. No items should ever be stored directly on a floor.

13.2.8 Sterile components should not be used beyond one working session.

13.2.9 Consumables used within the critical environment, EU GMP Grades A and B (EC 2015), should be sterile.

13.2.10 Once transferred into the clean room using the spray and wipe technique, paper-backed components should not be stored in the clean room (see Chapter 12: Cleaning, sanitisation and biodecontamination).

References

British Standards Institute (BSI) (2012). *BS EN ISO 13485:2012 Medical Devices: Quality Management Systems, requirements for regulatory purposes.* London: BSI.

Department of Health (DH) (2013). Health Technical Memorandum CFPP 01-01. *Decontamination of surgical instruments.* Available at: **https://www.gov.uk/government/publications/management-and-decontamination-of-surgical-instruments-used-in-acute-care** (accessed 14 April 2016).

European Commission (2015). *The rules governing medicinal products in the European Community. Vol IV. Good Manufacturing Practice for medicinal products.* Available at: **http://ec.europa.eu/health/documents/eudralex/vol-4/index_en.htm** (accessed 26 February 2016).

Institute of Sterile Services Management (ISSM) (2000). *CSSD – Quality Standards and Recommended Practices for Sterile Services Departments.* Truro: Institute of Sterile Services Management.

Medicines and Healthcare products Regulatory Agency (MHRA) (2014). *The supply of unlicensed medicinal products ("specials").* MHRA Guidance Note 14. London: Medicines and Healthcare products Regulatory Agency. Available at: **https://www.gov.uk/government/publications/supply-unlicensed-medicinal-products-specials** (accessed 15 April 2016).

NHS Pharmaceutical Quality Assurance Committee (PQAC) (2014). *Vial Sharing in Aseptic Services.* NHS Pharmaceutical Quality Assurance Committee. Available at: **www.medicinesresources.nhs.uk/en/Communities/NHS/UKQAInfoZone/National-resources/NHSPQA-Committee-/NHSPQA-Yellow-Cover-Guidance/Vial-Sharing-in-Aseptic-Services-Edition-1-August-2014/** (accessed 02 September 2015).

CHAPTER 14 PRODUCT APPROVAL

Units operate under a professional exemption to the UK *Medicines Act 1968* and incorporated into the *Human Medicines Regulations 2012*. This allows preparation of pharmaceuticals to be undertaken without the need for product and manufacturing licences to be held. Supervision, as applied to Section 10 aseptic preparation activities, has been defined by the NHS (PQAC 2014). This definition cannot be considered in isolation and should be fully supported by the UK national competency framework for product approval (ASAWG 2014) giving assurance of resource, governance and oversight in line with national requirements.

14.1 A formal, recorded decision of product approval (release) should be taken by an Accredited Product Approver before a product is released and after completion of all preparation and checking procedures. (Use of a checklist may be helpful for complex products).

14.2 The Accountable Pharmacist should ensure that robust systems are in place to train, assess and authorise individuals to carry out the product approval process. For non-pharmacists, these systems should comply with the UK national competency framework for product approval (ASAWG 2014) requirements. A current list of Accredited Product Approvers should be available.

14.3 The Accountable Pharmacist should ensure that an effective and comprehensive Pharmaceutical Quality System is in place within the unit (see Chapter 8: Pharmaceutical Quality System).

14.4 There should be an appropriate structure so that all Accredited Product Approvers are accountable directly to the Accountable Pharmacist for this activity and that this is reflected in their job description.

14.5 The Accredited Product Approver should not, other than in exceptional circumstances, be the person who prepared the product.

Note: Out of hours the requirements for supervision still apply.

14.6 There should be written procedures covering final accuracy checking and product approval (release). These processes may, or may not, be undertaken by the same person. Details of the roles and responsibilities of all the staff involved in these processes should be clearly defined.

14.7　The Authorised Pharmacist responsible for supervision should be identifiable and contactable at any point.

14.8　The Accredited Product Approver should ensure that they are authorised to approve the specific product for release, e.g. cytotoxics, parenteral nutrition etc.

Note: Intrathecal chemotherapy should only be approved for release by an Authorised Pharmacist named on the intrathecal chemotherapy register (DH 2008).

14.9　All those involved in the process of product approval should maintain the appropriate levels of competence and act in accordance with the GPhC standards of conduct, ethics and performance (GPhC 2015).

14.10　The Accredited Product Approver should, after completion of the preparation process but before release:

■ carry out a visual inspection of the product (for particles, precipitation and integrity)

■ ensure that the product complies with the prescription, the clinical trial protocol (if applicable) and the appropriate specification, including labelling

■ ensure that the product has been prepared by competent and validated operators according to approved procedures, and be aware of any deviation reports

■ be aware of recent microbiological and environmental results for the facilities

■ ensure that the daily monitoring records for the unit are satisfactory, e.g. pressure differentials, cleaning

■ be aware of the status of the unit and ensure the planned preventative maintenance programme is up to date

■ be aware of recent retrospective testing results for products

■ consider any prospective testing results, e.g. analytical testing, weight checks

■ ensure that all necessary accuracy checks e.g. including in-process checks and reconciliation of empty and part-used containers of starting materials have been carried out

■ ensure any planned deviations (temporary change controls) have been approved by an Authorised Pharmacist.

14.11   In the case of any unplanned deviation, any decision to approve the product should be taken by an Authorised Pharmacist.

14.12   All errors detected should be recorded via the Pharmaceutical Aseptic Services Group (PASG) national aseptic error reporting scheme, or the UK Radiopharmacy Group error reporting scheme (if appropriate). They should be trended and investigated to an appropriate level depending upon the severity.

14.13   The Authorised Pharmacist should be aware of, and act on, any errors detected and any interventions made both during the preparative stages and/ or at the product approval stage. This is relevant even where the product is able to be released.

14.14   There should be a written procedure for dealing with preparations failing to meet the required standard. The investigation of these events should be fully documented and corrective and/or preventative actions (CAPA) implemented to an appropriate level. Trending of failures should be undertaken regularly and any adverse trends or major failures to comply with standards should be brought to the attention of the Chief Pharmacist (see Chapter 5: Management).

References

Department of Health (DH) (2008). *Updated National Guidance on Safe Administration of Intrathecal Chemotherapy.* HSC 2008/001. London: Department of Health.

General Pharmaceutical Council (GPhC) (2015). *Standards of conduct, ethics and performance.* Available at: **https://www.pharmacyregulation.org/standards/conduct-ethics-and-performance** (accessed 26 February 2016)

Medicines Act 1968, c67. London: HMSO. Available at: **http://www.legislation.gov.uk/ukpga/1968/67** (accessed 26 February 2016)

NHS Aseptic Services Accreditations Working Group (ASAWG) (2014). *Nationally Recognised Competency Framework for Pharmacists and Pharmacy Technicians: Product Approval (Release) in Aseptic Services under Section 10 Exemption.* Available at: **www.nhspedc.nhs.uk/supports.htm** (accessed 25 February 2016).

NHS Pharmaceutical Quality Assurance Committee (PQAC) (2014). *Guidance on the Definition of Supervision as Applied to Section 10 Aseptic Preparation Activities.*

The Human Medicines Regulations 2012. SI 2012 No. 1916. Available at: **www.legislation.gov.uk/uksi/2012/1916/contents/made** (accessed 26 February 2016).

Note:

At the time of publication there are currently consultations on:

■ The GPhC's *Standards of conduct, ethics and performance.* Details are available at: **https://www.pharmacyregulation.org/news/pharmacy-regulator-launches-major-consultation-new-standards-pharmacy-professionals** (accessed on 28 April 2016). Consultation closes 27 June 2016.

■ Changes to Section 10 of the *Medicines Act 1968.* This includes a proposal for the relevant provisions to appear in the *Human Medicines Regulations 2012.* Department of Health (2016). Pharmacy dispensing models and displaying prices on medicines. Available at: **https://www.gov.uk/government/consultations/pharmacy-dispensing-models-and-displaying-prices-on-medicines** (accessed on 28 April 2016). Consultation closes 17 May 2016.

CHAPTER 15 STORAGE AND DISTRIBUTION

With changes to NHS structures and the amalgamation of some hospitals into single entity, multi-sited bodies; storage and distribution of aseptically-prepared products assumes a higher priority than previously. Aseptic units performing any distribution activities are required to comply with the principles of Good Distribution Practice (GDP) (Guidelines on Good Distribution Practice of Medicinal Products for Human Use 2013) (EC 2013).

15.1 General issues

15.1.1 Staff involved with storage and distribution should be aware of their responsibilities with regard to the integrity of the product. Training and assessment should be undertaken as appropriate and the results documented (see Chapter 9: Personnel, training and competency assessment).

15.1.2 A close examination should be made of all stages between product approval and product use to ensure that the quality of the product is not compromised before its expiry.

15.2 Storage

15.2.1 Special attention should be paid to the storage of products with specific handling instructions as specified in national legislation. Special storage conditions (and special authorisations) may be required for such products. Radioactive materials and other hazardous products, as well as products presenting special safety risks of fire or explosion (e.g. combustibles, flammable liquids), should be stored in one or more dedicated areas subject to local legislation and appropriate safety and security measures, e.g. *The Control of Substances Hazardous to Health Regulations 2002, The Ionising Radiations Regulations 1999.*

15.2.2 Products should be stored under refrigeration, normally 2–8°C, unless it would be detrimental to the product to do so. Refrigerators should not be overloaded. For products and starting materials where refrigeration is not appropriate, suitable storage conditions should be maintained to ensure no deterioration occurs.

15.2.3 All refrigerators and other areas used for the storage of aseptic products and starting materials within the pharmacy should be temperature mapped before use and at defined intervals.

15.2.4 Refrigerators and other storage areas should be continually monitored to ensure compliance with the appropriate temperature range; 2–8°C for refrigerators, and not more than 25°C for ambient areas. Temperature monitoring should also take place in the end-user department.

15.2.5 The temperature monitoring procedure should include action to be taken in the event of an out-of-specification reading and appropriate records of actions should be maintained. Trend monitoring should be performed regularly.

15.2.6 Calibration of temperature monitoring equipment should be carried out annually using a two-point check as a minimum. The calibration should be traceable to a national or international measurement standard.

15.2.7 Any automatic temperature monitoring system should be validated initially and also subsequently when appropriate (see Part B – 2.6).

15.2.8 Equipment repair, maintenance and calibration operations should be carried out in such a way that the quality of the medicinal products being stored is not compromised.

15.2.9 Alarm systems should be in place to provide alerts when there are excursions from pre-defined storage conditions. Alarm levels should be appropriately set and alarms should be regularly tested to ensure adequate functionality. The Authorised Pharmacist supervising at the time should be aware of any alarms being activated and take appropriate action.

15.2.10 Should failure of refrigeration or cold chain occur for a limited period, for whatever reason, an informed decision on the continued viability of affected stock should be made from knowledge of the ambient temperature stability or consulting the manufacturer of the starting materials.

15.2.11 Any returned or unused products should be clearly marked and segregated from other products.

15.3 Distribution

15.3.1 Regardless of the method of distribution, products should not be exposed to conditions that may compromise their quality, security and integrity.

15.3.2 Distribution should be controlled and validated as rigorously as storage. Medicinal products should be transported in containers that have no adverse effect on the quality of the products, and that offer adequate protection from external influences, including seasonal variations in temperature, contamination etc.

15.3.3 Transit containers should be of an appropriate defined specification and comply with any appropriate regulations. (*Transport of Dangerous Goods (Safety Advisers) Regulations 1999, Carriage of Dangerous Goods by Road (Driver Training) Regulations 1996, The Carriage of Dangerous Goods and Use of Transportable Pressure Equipment Regulations 2009* (CDG 2009) and subsequent amendments.) Selection of a container and packaging should be based on the storage and transportation requirements of the medicinal products; the space required for the amount of medicines; the anticipated external temperature extremes; the estimated maximum time for transportation.

15.3.4 Due regard should be given to health and safety considerations relating to potential hazards posed by the products during distribution. All applicable regulations, e.g. *The Control of Substances Hazardous to Health Regulations 2002* and transport regulations (*Transport of Dangerous Goods (Safety Advisers) Regulations 1999, Carriage of Dangerous Goods by Road (Driver Training) Regulations 1996, The Carriage of Dangerous Goods and Use of Transportable Pressure Equipment Regulations 2009* (CDG 2009) and subsequent amendments), should be complied with. The hospital's safety advisor should be able to provide additional information.

15.3.5 Transit containers should bear labels providing sufficient information on handling and storage requirements and precautions to ensure that the products are properly handled and secured at all times. The containers should enable identification of the contents of the containers and the source.

15.3.6 Labelling on transit containers of potentially hazardous products (e.g. cytotoxics) should include details of contacts and actions to be taken in an emergency. For radiopharmaceuticals separate regulations apply. (*Transport of Dangerous Goods (Safety Advisers) Regulations 1999, Carriage of Dangerous Goods by Road (Driver Training) Regulations 1996, The Carriage of Dangerous Goods and Use of Transportable Pressure Equipment Regulations 2009* (CDG 2009) and subsequent amendments.)

15.3.7 Consideration should be given to preventing the relative movement of components, such as syringe barrel and plunger, during transport and storage.

15.3.8 Where appropriate, the security of the cold/ambient chain should be assured and periodically revalidated.

15.3.9 Staff involved in storage and distribution should be aware of their responsibilities with regard to the integrity of the product. Training and assessment should be undertaken as appropriate and the results documented.

15.3.10 Records should be maintained of the destination of all products if not recorded elsewhere, e.g. on the prescription. There should be additional recording systems for distribution of Controlled Drugs and radioactive products.

15.3.11 There should be a policy for the handling of returned or unused products, including any outsourced products, which considers environmental factors. Returned or unused products may be useful for testing purposes (see Chapter 11: Monitoring).

15.4 Complaints and recall

15.4.1 Complaints should be recorded with all the original details. A distinction should be made between complaints related to the quality of a medicinal product and those related to service, including distribution.

15.4.2 Any product complaint should be thoroughly investigated to identify the origin of, or reason for, the complaint. A person should be given specific responsibility for handling of complaints and allocated sufficient resource to satisfactorily discharge this responsibility.

15.4.3 If necessary, appropriate follow-up actions (including corrective and/ or preventative actions (CAPA)) should be taken after investigation and evaluation of the complaint.

15.4.4 Procedures for recall should be in place, and should be reviewed on a regular basis. These should cover the recall of products made by the aseptic unit in the event of a potential problem with the product itself or a known problem with any components or starting materials used in it, e.g. a Drug Alert issued either by MHRA or company-led, a Field Safety Notice for a component etc.

15.4.5 Recall exercises should be undertaken on an annual basis to ensure the efficiency and timeliness of the process, if an actual recall has not occurred. A report should be produced following assessment of the recall process (either through a simulated or actual recall).

QUALITY ASSURANCE OF ASEPTIC PREPARATION SERVICES:
STANDARDS HANDBOOK PART A

References

European Commission (2013). *Guidelines on Good Distribution Practice of Medicinal Products for Human Use* (2013/EC 343/01). November 2013. OJEU.

The Carriage of Dangerous Goods by Road (Driver Training) Regulations 1996. SI 1996 No. 2094. London: The Stationery Office.

The Carriage of Dangerous Goods and Use of Transportable Pressure Equipment Regulations 2009 (CDG 2009) and subsequent amendments. SI 2009 No. 1348. London: The Stationery Office.

The Carriage of Dangerous Goods and Use of Transportable Pressure Equipment (Amendment) Regulations 2011. SI 2011 No. 1885. London: The Stationery Office.

The Control of Substances Hazardous to Health Regulations (COSHH) 2002. SI 2002 No. 2677. London: The Stationery Office. Available at: **www.legislation.gov.uk/uksi/2002/2677/pdfs/uksi_20022677_en.pdf** (accessed 04 February 2016).

The Ionising Radiations Regulations 1999. SI 1999 No.3232. London: The Stationery Office.

Transport of Dangerous Goods (Safety Advisors) Regulations 1999. SI 1999 No. 257. London: The Stationery Office.

United Nations Economic Commission for Europe. *European Agreement concerning the International Carriage of Dangerous Goods by Road (ADR 2015).* Available at: **http://www.unece.org/trans/danger/publi/adr/adr2015/15contentse.html** (accessed 08 April 2016).

CHAPTER 16 INTERNAL AND EXTERNAL AUDIT

Systems need constant monitoring to ensure that they continue to meet the requirements and needs of the organisation.

A comprehensive programme of internal audits, undertaken by trained personnel, is essential to the continued effectiveness and further development of the Pharmaceutical Quality System (PQS). Internal audits can be used to identify system deficiencies, areas of non conformance and opportunities for improvement and should be programmed according to importance of the areas or processes being audited.

Internal audits (if undertaken conscientiously) provide those most familiar with the operation of the aseptic unit the opportunity to critique their processes as the auditors should be familiar with any perceived weak points in their operation. Internal audit, undertaken in a diligent manner, is therefore a fundamental part of Quality Management.

Results from both internal and external audits form an essential input into the management review process.

16.1 Audit involving all areas in which aseptic preparation takes place (including any satellites) should be undertaken on a regular planned basis (PQCC 1999) to monitor implementation and compliance with these defined NHS standards and to propose any corrective measures.

16.2 In addition to inspection of premises, equipment and processes, a detailed quality review of the Pharmaceutical Quality System (PQS) is required (see Chapter 8: Pharmaceutical Quality System).

16.3 The audit programme should be determined in advance with the plan documented and adhered to. A number of different techniques may be used. For example, low level regular housekeeping audits, higher level process audits such as horizontal audits or linear audits on a rotating programme and systems/checklist style audits on a less frequent basis (PQCC 1999).

16.4 Audits should include a review of the capacity planning within the unit (see Chapter 5: Management and Part B – 5).

16.5 Internal audit should be conducted in an independent and detailed way by designated and competent staff.

16.6 Observations made during audits should be clearly recorded along with any proposals for corrective actions.

16.7 An action plan should be drawn up detailing timescales and persons responsible for the actions.

16.8 There should be an SOP in place that details the management and review of the action plan, and the effectiveness of these procedures should be verified during audit. (See Chapter 5: Management and Chapter 8: Pharmaceutical Quality System).

16.9 Corrective actions should be reviewed at the next audit or earlier if appropriate.

16.10 The audit report should be submitted to senior management. Any deficiencies should be assessed in terms of risk to the quality of the product, and a decision to cease activity made if necessary. There should be appropriate escalation procedures in place allowing risks to be identified to the hospital management via the Chief Pharmacist.

16.11 An external audit should be carried out by the Regional Quality Assurance Specialist or any other accredited auditor (PQAC 2011) at least every 12 to 18 months (NHS Executive 1997). The unit should respond with a realistic action plan within the timeframe agreed with the auditor. Equivalent external audits are required in other Home Countries of the UK.

16.12 Aseptic units which prepare intrathecal chemotherapy should be subject to audits for compliance with the current *National Guidance on the Safe Administration of Intrathecal Chemotherapy* (DH 2008).

References

Department of Health (DH) (2008). *Updated National Guidance on Safe Administration of Intrathecal Chemotherapy.* HSC 2008/001. London: Department of Health.

NHS Executive (1997). *Executive Letter (97) 52: Aseptic Dispensing in NHS Hospitals.* London: Department of Health.

NHS Pharmaceutical Quality Assurance Committee (PQAC) (2011). *The Training of Auditors to Undertake Audits of Unlicensed Aseptic Dispensing in NHS Hospitals.* Edition 2.

NHS Pharmaceutical Quality Control Committee (PQCC) (1999). *Quality Audits and their Application to Hospital Pharmacy Technical Services.* Norwich: PQCC.

PART B – I: MICROBIOLOGICAL ENVIRONMENTAL MONITORING TECHNIQUES FOR THE LABORATORY

1.1 Introduction

The aim of this support resource is to provide guidance on the laboratory aspects of microbiological environmental monitoring in clean rooms and to facilitate the interpretation of microbiological monitoring results.

Microbiological monitoring standards and the programme and frequency of testing are described in Part A, Chapter 11.

This support resource encompasses the specification, supply and storage of growth media. It also provides advice on equipment, methods and individual techniques relevant to the detection, recovery, incubation, reading and interpretation of results. This is not exhaustive and other validated procedures are not precluded.

1.2 Terminology and abbreviations

TERM OR ABBREVIATION	DESCRIPTION
Bioburden	Degree of microbial contamination or microbial load; the number of microorganisms contaminating an object
cfu	Colony forming unit
Commensal	Harmless organism living in or with host to obtain food
FTM	Fluid Thioglycollate Medium BP
Genus (pl. Genera)	Family of organisms containing one or more species (for example, *Staphylococcus*, *Pseudomonas* etc.)
Medium	Liquid or gel designed to support the growth of microorganisms
Neutraliser	A chemical agent included in the formulation to counteract the effect of any inhibitory substances, for example, disinfectants

TERM OR ABBREVIATION	DESCRIPTION
Objectionable organism	Organisms which may be hazardous/pathogenic to a specific patient or patient group (MHRA 2015)
Opportunistic pathogen	Organism that may live harmlessly on a host until circumstances change, allowing the organism to take up a pathogenic role, i.e. wounds, compromised immune system etc.
Pathogen	Organism causing disease
Saprophyte	Organism living on dead or decaying organic matter
SDA	Sabouraud Dextrose Agar BP
sp.	One species of genus isolated (for example, *Staphylococcus sp.*)
Species	Specific organism within a genus, for example, *Staphylococcus aureus*, *Pseudomonas aeruginosa*
spp.	More than one species of genus isolated
Sterile	Free from microorganisms
Sterility Assurance Level	Is the probability of a single unit being non-sterile after it has been subjected to sterilisation
Strain	A genetic variant or subtype of a microorganism species
TSA	Tryptone Soya Agar BP
TSB	Tryptone Soya Broth BP

1.3 Facilities

Standards for facilities processing microbiological samples are described in Part A, Chapter 7.

1.4 General considerations applicable to the specific techniques

1.4.1 Media and reagents

Media and reagents should be purchased, where possible, ready prepared and sterile from a supplier experienced in pharmaceutical microbiology. They should be accompanied by a Certificate of Analysis (CofA) for each batch which includes chemical composition, pH, fertility and sterility statements. Appropriate neutralisers may also be present where required. Together these form the basis of a specification for the medium.

Where media are made in-house, all appropriate verifications for the above factors should be applied and documented.

Media should be stored according to the manufacturer's instructions, protected from light and in the original packaging.

Each container (such as a settle plate or broth bottle) should be individually labelled with the description of the culture medium, storage conditions, batch number and expiry date by the supplier. Labels should not interfere with the ability to detect and read growth.

The control of temperature and light is very difficult between the point of manufacture and the point of use. CofAs cannot be relied upon to ensure the media or reagents are fit for purpose at the time of use. Positive and negative controls are required to verify the fertility of batches of the media before use. There should be a validated shelf life assigned to each product (a batch at the end of its shelf life could be periodically sent back to the manufacturer for fertility testing). It is advised that a simple growth promotion test is conducted. For example, a positive control plate can be exposed in an uncontrolled environment for 4 hours and deemed to have passed if more than 5 colony forming units (cfu) per plate are recovered. A negative control plate should similarly be left, but not exposed, and deemed to have passed if no growth is recovered.

1.4.2 Solid media (agar): general consideration

Solid media (settle plates, contact plates, agar strips etc.) should be purchased double- or triple-wrapped and irradiated to give a sterility assurance of at least 10^{-6}. It is expected that media suppliers will have been audited by the NHS so audit reports should, therefore, be available for review. This removes the requirement for pre-incubation to demonstrate sterility of the batch before use.

Note: The volume of fill of settle plates should be sufficient to prevent drying out (equivalent to less than 20% weight loss of the media), typically in excess of 20ml in a 90mm petri dish. For contact plates, the fill should be sufficient to maintain an integral raised surface throughout its shelf life.

Plates should be stored in the inverted position, to reduce the risk of condensation falling onto the agar surface.

During storage, wide fluctuations in temperature should be avoided to minimise condensation and deterioration resulting in the loss of fertility. Similarly, plates should be packaged to minimise the build up of condensation and allow air to permeate.

Refrigeration of plates before use is not generally recommended as the dew point could be exceeded, resulting in condensation. If plates have been refrigerated before use, it is advisable to allow warming to room temperature before exposure.

Before use in environmental monitoring, it is essential that media are checked for contamination, desiccation and excessive condensation.

The inner wrap of sessional settle plates and finger dabs should be removed in the critical zone. Plates used other than in the critical zone should have the inner wrap removed in the area to be monitored.

Note: Unused plates can be transferred for use in lower grade areas.

Sampling should be in accordance with a pre-determined site plan designed at the qualification of the facility and that represents the best chance of detecting any microorganisms generated from the work activity. All samples should be labelled to clearly indicate the area concerned, in compliance with this plan. Details on the plate should be sufficient to show operator, site, location, date and time exposed. In the case of agar plates, the ideal place to label is on the base of the dish. (Generally, paper labels are best avoided as they can become detached, obscure vision and may be a source of extraneous contamination.)

1.4.3 Selection of agar

There is no single agar formulation available to allow the growth of all microorganisms at the same temperature in a short period of time. Selective agars have been developed for the growth of a particular genus or species but these are not generally used to monitor aseptic preparation. The agar should be stable enough to permit sterilisation by gamma irradiation.

Note: The typical gamma irradiation sterilisation dose of 25 kilogray (kGy) may give rise to poor performance unless the formulation is modified. (The supplier should be aware of this.) The majority of monitoring is based on Tryptone Soya Agar (TSA). Some laboratories use Tryptone Soya plus Glucose Agar (TSA+G) to encourage the growth of bacteria and fungi on a single plate at a single temperature. Evidence is available to support this (Rhodes et al 2016).

If TSA plates are incubated at 30-35°C, it is desirable to incorporate a proactive component in the monitoring schedule to detect moulds and yeasts, which should be incubated at a lower temperature.

A selective medium that supports fungal growth would ideally be incorporated into the schedule of monitoring; for example, TSA+G or Sabouraud Dextrose Agar (SDA):

- SDA settle plates used monthly within the unit, and/or
- SDA active air (strips/plates) samples used monthly within the unit.

TSA settle plates should be critically examined for yeasts and moulds and enumerated separately from bacteria. Where fungal contamination is detected at levels which cause concern, either from SDA or TSA monitoring, additional SDA plates or swabs should be instigated to further evaluate the situation. The prevalence of conditions which promote fungal contamination (for example, humidity, dust from building work) should trigger additional monitoring. Additional monitoring is, however, never a substitute for the prospective implementation of steps taken to minimise the spread of contamination. To reduce the risk of contamination ingress into microbiologically controlled areas, an additional sporicidal wipe of items into an inner support room may be useful under these circumstances.

Alternative media are permitted provided they have been validated using both a range of standard strains of microorganisms, as well as microorganisms from the environment to be monitored.

1.4.4 Transportation and sample receipt

It is essential that, during sampling, handling and transport, all possible sources of extraneous contamination are excluded. For this reason, plates should be secured, labelled and packaged appropriately for transport in the cleanest practical area.

During transportation, the effects of vibration should be minimised. In addition, efforts should be made to ensure that plates are carried inverted, i.e. the lids are at the bottom. This is to minimise false readings, for example due to the effects of condensation, such as colony spread. Where provided, locking lids should be used and engaged; where not available, some means of securing the lids to the base should be employed.

Agar plates should be despatched promptly for incubation. Delays should be avoided but, when necessary, plates are best held at ambient temperature (inverted) until transport is available. Refrigeration is not generally recommended, as this may inhibit recovery. Any storage should be validated and be for a minimal defined time (less than 7 days).

Where plates have to be transported, the worst case scenario process should be validated. During any transportation, plates should be protected from light, extremes of temperature and external contamination.

During incubation, plates which are wrapped too tightly (hermetically sealed) may engender excessive condensation, which can cause random multiplication of colony forming units (cfus) when changing temperature i.e. during incubation. The use of adhesive tape, parcel tape and similar materials are particularly prone to this problem. Where plastic bags are used, these should be either new or sterile.

Elastic bands to hold plates together are acceptable, but an overwrap is desirable, to prevent contamination from external sources during transit. Cling film has been found to be useful. If plates have been wrapped in cling film, there is no need to remove it until the time to read the plates.

Upon receipt into the laboratory, an assessment of the exposed plate condition and packaging should be made. Any cracked or broken plates (including damaged media) should be noted on the report form. Any mould growth outside a plate should be reported and the packaging and plate carefully removed from the stack and clean packaging applied to the remaining plates.

1.4.5 Incubation

Plates should be incubated in the inverted position, to reduce the risk of condensation falling onto the agar surface.

Movement of plates during incubation should be limited and carried out carefully to minimise spreading of colonies by spores or droplets, resulting in increased counts. This is particularly important when transferring plates from one incubator to another and/or carrying out an interim read.

The microbiological growth media judged to be acceptable for use in pharmaceutical aseptic preparation units are included in Table 1, below:

Table B1.1

Media used for routine settle plate environmental monitoring, active air sampling and finger dabs

MEDIA	USE	TYPICAL INCUBATION TEMPERATURE	MINIMUM INCUBATION PERIOD
Tryptone Soya Agar (TSA)	total bacterial count (this will also detect certain yeasts and moulds)	30-35°C	5 days (7 days recommended)
Sabouraud Dextrose Agar (SDA)	selective determination of yeasts and moulds	20-25°C	7 days (14 days recommended)
Tryptone Soya plus Glucose Agar (TSA+G)	combined detection of bacteria, yeasts and moulds	22.5-27.5°C	5 days (7 days recommended)

To avoid routinely using SDA plates and to minimise the number of invasive procedures in an aseptic clean room, many sites choose to use a standard general purpose medium e.g. TSA and employ a dual temperature incubation regime which allows the recovery of aerobic bacteria and fungi (yeasts and moulds).

Dual temperature incubation regimes employ a fixed, or minimum, period at one set temperature followed by a fixed, or minimum, period at a higher or lower temperature. A number of incubation regimes have been developed by NHS Quality Control (QC) laboratories, based on knowledge of the environment being monitored and local circumstances.

Most dual temperature regimes employ a period at 20-25°C and a period at 30-35°C, for example:

- Low-High Incubation e.g. 5 days at 20-25°C followed by 2 days at 30-35°C
- High-Low Incubation e.g. 2 days at 30-35°C followed by 5 days at 20-25°C.

The incubation time and temperature can also vary; some laboratories allocate equal time to each temperature range, for example 3 days at 20-25°C followed by 3 days at 30-35°C.

If the environment monitoring results suggest that fungal colonies may be present, the Low-High incubation regime is advised.

If fungal colonies are rarely detected and a bacterial monitoring result is required quickly, then the High-Low incubation regime can be recommended provided the periodic monitoring with a selective medium for fungi is also used so that any increase in fungal contamination can be detected and acted upon. (See 1.4.3).

Dual temperature incubation is often preferred when process validation, operator validation or end of session broth tests are incubated – see Sections 9 and 10.

2   Reading of results

Only staff with suitable training should be engaged in the reading and interpretation of microbiological test results.

Agar plates should be read in a good light that reveals both the numbers and morphological characteristics of colonies. A simple count of colony forming units (cfus) is the first step in interpreting the microbiological environmental results. It is important to distinguish at this stage between bacteria, moulds and yeasts. These should be recorded and reported.

It is important not to extrapolate results from small volumes obtained during active air sampling and small areas obtained during surface sampling to larger volumes/areas as this may produce misleading information especially in EU GMP Grades A and B (EC 2015) environments. Similarly, when plates have been exposed for less than the standard four hours, correction factors should be avoided.

It is important to ensure that sufficient information is available from the environmental monitoring programme to identify any loss of control in a timely manner to enable appropriate remedial actions.

The laboratory should have sufficient capacity to handle routine testing plates and the additional work generated during the qualification and validation of a new facility plus any additional monitoring required following an action limit being exceeded. In addition, there should be sufficient capacity to cope with incubator failures and cleaning.

Sufficient resource should be available to ensure that the cleaning and environmental monitoring programme is sustainable.

2.1   Identification of isolates: general considerations

All microorganisms recovered exceeding the action limits, or from sterility test and broth test failures, should be identified. The information should be used to determine the best course of action to allow aseptic services staff to deal with the contamination and return the unit to control. Identification to genus level should allow the correct action to be taken, whilst identification of species assists with determining the likely source. Further identification of an organism strain is not appropriate for routine environmental monitoring, but can be useful for investigating a sterility or broth test failure.

2.2   Basic identification of microorganisms

It is possible for experienced staff to visually identify some colonies as a first indicator of identity; for example, colonies suggestive of *Staphylococcus, Bacillus* or *Penicillium*. An alternative approach is by comparison to an in-house reference file, which may include photographs of the macroscopic appearance of known organisms on the agar used and other information to aid identification. The staff performing visual microorganism identification should be able to demonstrate adequate training and experience (see Section 3).

Identification of microorganisms to genus level is normally sufficient to trigger appropriate control measures and a response should be initiated in a timely manner rather than waiting for species identification.

A list of commonly-found organisms for a unit is a useful reference point to determine whether an isolate is unusual and requires further investigation.

If visual identification is inconclusive, or there is not enough information in the reference file, the following should be carried out by trained and experienced personnel.

Basic tests that should be routinely carried out:

- Colony morphology
- Gram stain
- Microscopy
- Odour.

If necessary, the following tests can be utilised to provide further definition:

- Oxidase enzymatic tests
- Catalase enzymatic tests
- Coagulase enzymatic tests
- KOH String test
- Malachite green test
- Motility assessment.

More detailed information on the procedures for the identification of microorganisms is given in Section 3.

2.2.1 The Gram stain is used in identification of bacteria and should be performed with 18-24 hour cultures. It is recommended that the flow chart is followed to identify organisms isolated.

2.2.2 Bacteria can be divided into two main groups, Gram-positive and Gram-negative. After staining following the procedure outlined in Section 3.2, Gram-positive bacteria appear purple and Gram-negative bacteria appear pink/red, when observed microscopically. Some organisms such as *Corynebacterium variabilis* are Gram-variable by displaying purple and pink colouration. Some organisms, such as *Bacillus*, lose some of their cell wall properties with age or following treatment with bactericidal agents and appear to be Gram-negative. The flow chart Figure B1.1, can be used to guide subsequent tests to narrow the identification.

2.2.3 Moulds are identified using a separate technique, as outlined in Figure B1.1 and Section 3.8.

It is essential that, for all confirmatory tests, only pure culture is used. If a high level of background flora is observed on the agar plate, the colony may be streaked out to isolation using a purity streak.

Figure B1.1
Organism identification flowchart

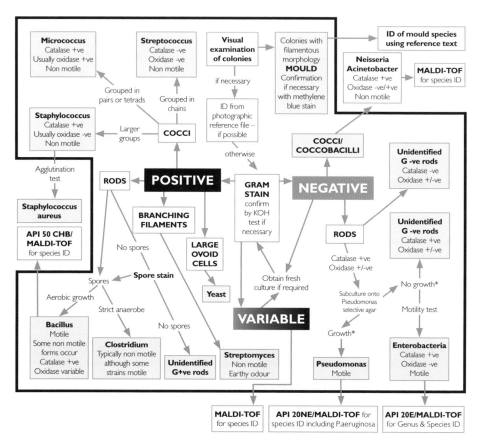

Only statements in bold in light blue boxes may be reported.
Statements outside the dark blue line are optional tests/IDs to be performed when directed by Section Head Microbiology.
*It is possible that Enterobacteria are capable of growing on Pseudomonas selective agar.

QUALITY ASSURANCE OF ASEPTIC PREPARATION SERVICES:
STANDARDS HANDBOOK PART B

3 Traditional phenotypic procedure for identification of microorganisms

3.1 The staff performing visual microorganism identification should be able to demonstrate adequate training and experience. This can be achieved by a regular programme of genus testing organisms which have been previously identified, preferably down to species level. It is recommended that staff take part in the process, with a minimum of one check per person per quarter using a range of organisms.

3.1.1 Organisms isolated in EU GMP Grade A (EC 2015) and, in certain circumstances, EU GMP Grade B (EC 2015) areas should be identified to species level (see Section 3.9). Organisms isolated in EU GMP Grade B (EC 2015) (in normal circumstances), C and D (EC 2015) areas should be counted, unless the count exceeds an action limit, at which point identification to genus level is required. Organisms isolated in areas outside the classified zones should be counted and, where appropriate, identified to genus level.

3.1.2 It is important that any identification is based on pure cultures, particularly with biochemical tests. Where necessary the colonies should be subcultured to provide a pure and viable culture (when subculturing, samples should be taken from the growing edge of the colony). If a culture is more than 18-24 hours old, further sub culture may be necessary to ensure appropriate reaction with the Gram stain or counter stain, or when identification using Matrix Assisted Laser Desorption/Ionisation – Time of Flight (MALDI-TOF) is employed.

3.1.3 The organism can be identified visually by comparison to an in-house reference file, which may include photographs of macroscopic appearance and information to aid identification. If there is not enough information in the reference file, Gram staining with microscopy should be used to enhance identification. Information is available to aid identification, for example, *Cowan and Steel's Manual for the Identification of Medical Bacteria* (Barrow and Feltham 2003).

3.1.4 Spore stains, catalase, oxidase, coagulase and motility tests are also used to assist in the identification of microorganisms.

3.1.5 Moulds are identified using a separate technique, see Section 3.8.

3.2 Gram stain

The Gram stain differentiates bacteria, based on their cell wall structure. Gram-positive organisms retain the crystal violet and iodine complex after being exposed to decolourising solution whereas Gram-negative bacteria do not. Safranin acts as a counterstain, staining all bacteria, allowing easier differentiation between Gram-positive and Gram-negative cells. An example of a suitable method is detailed below.

3.2.1 Preparation of a slide

1   Collect a glass microscope slide and, if necessary, sterilise by holding in forceps and passing through a Bunsen burner flame. Write the laboratory reference number of the sample requiring identification on the slide, using a diamond-tip pencil, or other equivalent indelible marker.

2   Sterilise an inoculating loop by heating in the Bunsen flame and use it to transfer two loopfuls of water or saline onto the slide.

3   Sterilise the inoculating loop again, cool, and use it to remove a small section from the edge of a single colony of the culture to be identified from the agar plate, being careful to avoid too heavy an inoculum.

4   Mix the colony into the water on the slide and, using the straight wire of the loop, spread the mixture in a thin film evenly over the slide.

5   The slide should then preferably be air dried. If necessary, to speed the process up, the slide may be placed into an incubator set at 25-37°C or alternatively, placed under a Bunsen flame by holding the slide with forceps and gently heating the slide culture side up under the Bunsen flame. It is imperative that the slide is not overheated as this may cause damage to the cells' structure. When the culture mixture is dry, fix, by passing quickly through the Bunsen flame twice. Alternatively, use a hot plate technique to dry and fix the stain.

6   Place the slide on the staining rack above the sink and allow to cool.

3.2.2 Staining

1   Apply Gram's crystal violet solution to the slide, flooding with the stain so that there are no gaps, and leave for 1-2 minutes. Holding with forceps, wash under slow-running, cold tap water. Ensure washing at this stage is not excessive.

2   Place the slide back on the staining rack. Apply Gram's iodine, flooding the slide as before and leave for 1-2 minutes. Wash under slow-running, cold tap water.

3   Holding the slide with the forceps, apply alcohol/acetone decolourising solution to the wet slide. This stage is critical and the decolouriser should only be left on for 5-10 seconds. Rinse again with running, cold tap water and place the slide on the rack.

4   Apply safranin counter stain, flooding the slide for 1-2 minutes. Wash under running cold tap water.

5   Blot the slide and allow to air dry. Transfer to the microscope for viewing.

3.2.3 Results

When viewed microscopically, Gram-positive bacteria appear as purple/blue and Gram-negative bacteria are red/pink. The Gram stain result is extremely important because it is used as the first stage in identification and many microbes become Gram-variable as they age. It is, therefore, possible for a Gram-positive organism to give a Gram-negative result as the culture ages. If any doubt exists, the culture should be re-streaked and re-stained the following day. The KOH String test can also be used to confirm the Gram stain result (see Section 3.7). If the stain has been performed correctly it is not possible for Gram-negative bacteria to give a Gram-positive result.

3.3   Spore stain

An example of a suitable method is detailed below:

1   The spore stain is used to reveal bacterial spores not easily visible without staining. The sample organism should be subjected to environmental stress, such as nutrient deprivation or cold shock refrigeration, to produce the metabolically inactive or dormant form called an endospore. (For example, refrigerate the plate for at least six hours, or a sample on a slide for 1-2 hours; this should be validated locally.) Prepare the slide as for Gram stain and place on the staining rack.

2   Flood the slide with malachite green. Heat the underneath of the slide, carefully using a Bunsen burner, until the slide steams. Alternatively heat the slide over a beaker of boiling water. Leave to cool for 1-2 minutes. Repeat the heating as above. Wash the slide under running, cold tap water. Counterstain with safranin and blot with a paper towel and air dry.

3   Heating the slide drives fat-soluble malachite green into the bacterial spores. The safranin counter stain reveals the unstained bacterial cells.

4   Spores are stained green; bacterial cells have a pink colouration.

3.4 Catalase test

1   A clean microscope slide is required. Add one drop of sterile hydrogen peroxide 3% (10 volume) to the slide.

2   Using a sterilised inoculating loop, remove a colony to be identified and mix with the hydrogen peroxide solution. Production of gas bubbles in the mixture indicates a positive reaction for the catalase test. This reaction is usually immediate. If no gas bubbles are produced within sixty seconds, this is considered a negative reaction.

3.5 Oxidase test

1   Dispense 2ml of sterile distilled water into a clean test tube. Add a small amount (roughly 0.02g is sufficient) of tetramethyl-p-phenylene diamine dihydrochloride reagent into the tube and mix gently.

2   Pour a few drops of the prepared solution onto a suitable filter paper, being careful not to over saturate the paper.

3   Remove a single colony of the organism to be identified using a sterile disposable inoculating loop or other device. Rub gently onto the filter paper.

    Note: Nichrome loops may cause false positives. High levels of carbohydrate in agar may cause false negatives and blood agar may cause false positives.

4   The solution only has a working life of approximately one hour.

5   The test is positive for oxidase if a colour change to purple is observed within sixty seconds.

3.6 Coagulase test

The coagulase test can be used to help identify potential *Staphylococcus aureus* cultures, as most strains of *S. aureus* produce coagulase. The coagulase test can be carried out using either the rabbit plasma tube coagulase method, or using a commercially-available agglutination kit.

Instructions for carrying out the coagulase test using an agglutination kit are provided here. If the instructions here differ from the manufacturer's instructions, then follow the manufacturer's instructions.

1   A variety of coagulase kits are available, some of which test for coagulase production alone e.g. Staphylase™, and others which test for coagulase along with other features common to *S. aureus*, such as Protein A e.g. Staphaurex™ or Staphytect™. All kits that test for coagulase and include a control reagent to test for auto agglutination are acceptable.

2   Ensure the test kit is at room temperature and mixed well before use.

3   Put a drop of test reagent onto the reaction card provided. If using, put a separate drop of control reagent onto the card also.

4   Using a sterilised, inoculating loop, pick up a section of the culture and mix the colony into the test reagent. If provided, mix the same colony into the control reagent simultaneously, using a separate sterile loop.

5   Rock the suspension gently for the specified period of time (usually around twenty seconds or a minute).

6   A positive result is indicated by the test reagent agglutinating to form clear clumps in the suspension within the specified period of time. A negative result is indicated by no clumping of the reagent within the specified time. If used, the control reagent should not agglutinate.

7   It is important not to confuse negative granular or stringy reactions for a positive result. Look at the manufacturer's instructions for more information and advice regarding interpretation of results.

8   Use of a positive and negative control alongside the test is recommended.

    Limitations: Not all strains of *S. aureus* produce coagulase and so would not react to form a positive result. Other species of bacteria can cause agglutination, so a Gram stain should be performed prior to testing to decrease the chances of this occurring. (See individual kit instructions for more information.)

3.7   KOH String test

The KOH String test is another method for distinguishing Gram-positive from Gram-negative bacteria and should be used when the Gram stain result is unclear.

1   Add a drop of 3% potassium hydroxide (KOH) solution to a clean sterile microscopic slide.

2   Using a sterilised inoculating loop, remove a section of the colony to be identified and mix with the potassium hydroxide solution.

3   Mix and then slowly lift the loop around 1-2cm above the slide. Gram-negative bacteria form a 'string' between the slide and loop when the loop is lifted. This should occur within sixty seconds of mixing. Gram-positive bacteria will not form this string within sixty seconds.

4   It is recommended that a positive and negative control should be run alongside the test to ensure the method is working effectively.

Note: It is important that a sufficient amount of culture is used for this test as, if not, this may lead to false negative (i.e. false Gram-positive) results.

3.8   Identification of moulds

If further identification to genus level is required, the following method may be used:

1   Prepare a microscope slide as detailed above. Add 1-2 drops of methylene blue to the slide.

2   Using a small piece of adhesive tape, remove a small amount of the colony. Press the adhesive tape onto the slide with the methylene blue and press down gently to remove any air bubbles.

3   An alternative to this method is to use two sterile, steel pins to carefully remove a small section of the colony, being careful not to disturb the structures. Transfer the colony onto a clean glass slide containing a small amount of sterile water or saline.

4   Examine the slide microscopically. If the structures are too highly disturbed using the adhesive tape method, use the steel pin method as an alternative. Identification is performed by reference to the appropriate mycological text (Barnett and Hunter 1987, Bridson 2002).

3.9   Identification of organisms to species level

If further identification is required, this may be performed to species level using the Analytical Profile Index (API) or similar biochemical system, following the manufacturer's instructions.

Identification should be to species level in the following circumstances:

Table B1.2

CIRCUMSTANCE	GUIDANCE
High individual counts	>5 cfu/session in EU GMP Grade B (EC 2015).
Trends	Trends greater than 5 cfu in 2 weeks in a EU GMP Grade B (EC 2015) environment should be investigated and the organism(s) identified to species level where possible.
Recovery of potentially objectionable organisms	Organisms which may be hazardous/pathogenic to a specific patient or patient group. When genus shows the organism to be 'objectionable', identification to species level is required.

In order to comply with the above expectation, it may be necessary to routinely retain all EU GMP Grade B (EC 2015) plates for two weeks to identify all organisms contributing to an adverse trend. The list of objectionable organisms is variable, and can include organisms from several genera. Best practice is to define the list of objectionable organisms for each site. (See also Sutton 2012.)

The development of instrument-based, rapid microbiological identification techniques offers cost effective and time efficient identification. However, it is necessary to ensure these techniques are appropriately validated and the instruments maintained to ensure reliable results. The development of specialist databases, particularly relating to environmental organisms, has made this more useful. These include:

Table B1.3

Vitek™	An automated biochemical system often used for clinical purposes.
MALDI-TOF	This equipment can also be used to identify moulds and yeasts to species level. Usage has grown, however, an environmental organism database is required for pharmaceutical use.
PCR (Polymerase Chain Reaction)	An amplification method employed to assist genotypic methods which can be used to identify strains.
RNA/DNA bacterial sequencing	A genotypic method.

4   Laboratory equipment

Equipment used in monitoring, for example in active air sampling, should be calibrated at least annually to ensure that the item is within specification with regard to efficiency and volume of sampling.

Incubators should be continually monitored for temperature by a method which allows the time out of specification to be determined and for an alarm to be raised when out of specification. As with all temperature controlled areas, a temperature-mapping exercise should be conducted at least every three to five years, or after any significant change in the equipment or monitoring results. Particular attention should be given to matching the routine temperature probes with the mapping data.

There are significant benefits to having an on-call system employing staff that have been trained to understand the significance of temperature excursions.

Clean rooms and clean air devices used for sterility testing should be controlled and maintained in accordance with Good Manufacturing Practice (GMP) standards, refer to Part A, Chapters 7, 8, 9, 11 and 12.

Equipment used to test samples or identify organisms should be validated and maintained via an appropriate contract. Consumables should be controlled as described in Part A, Chapter 13.

5   Active air sampling

5.1   Centrifugal

5.1.1   Materials

Centrifugal sampling equipment is available from a number of suppliers, for example, Biotest. The equipment uses special plastic strips containing agar. Gamma irradiated strips in packs of five are preferred. A limited range of agars are available and include:

- TSA for aerobic bacteria
- SDA for yeasts and moulds.

5.1.2 Technique

Ensure that the sampling head of the equipment is thoroughly disinfected (preferably sterilised by autoclaving) before use. Disinfect the outer wrapper of the strip before opening and pay particular attention to aseptic technique throughout. Open the outer wrapper and peel back the plastic seal a few centimetres, then remove the agar strip with the coated side facing downwards. Aseptically insert the strip into the impeller drum. Operate the sampler at the site.

Current guidelines (EC 2015) recommend a 1000 litre sample at each site. On completion of the sample, using aseptic technique remove the strip and replace it in its original wrapper, seal, label and return it to the laboratory for incubation and reading – see Sections 5.4 and Section 5.5.

5.2 Impaction

5.2.1 Materials

Equipment for active air sampling, using impaction onto an agar plate, is available from several manufacturers. The surface of the agar should be flat and the distance between the sieve and agar surface should be constant for each determination. The majority of manufacturers use 90mm settle plates, however, there is at least one manufacturer that uses 55mm contact plates.

The agar plates to be used should contain the same media as those employed in routine environmental monitoring.

5.2.2 Technique

Ensure that the sampling head of the equipment is thoroughly disinfected (preferably sterilised by autoclaving) before use. Carefully remove an agar plate from its sterile overwrap. Place the lidded plate in the sampler and remove the lid using aseptic technique. Operate the sampler at the site. Current guidelines (EC 2015) recommend a 1000 litre sample at each site. On completion, replace the lid on the plate, remove from sampler, seal, label and return it to the laboratory for incubation and reading – see Sections 5.4 and 5.5.

5.3 Gelatine filter impaction

5.3.1 Materials

The gelatine filter collection equipment is available from Sartorius (MD8). The media is supplied sterile in packs of fifty.

5.3.2 Technique

Ensure that the filter holder is thoroughly disinfected (preferably sterilised by autoclaving) prior to use. Disinfect the outer pack prior to the assembly of the gelatine filter into the holder.

Operate the sampler at the site. Current guidelines (EC 2015) recommend that 1000 litres of air is sampled at each site. On completion of the sample, using aseptic technique, transfer the filter directly onto the surface of an appropriate agar plate, seal, label and return it to the laboratory for incubation and reading – see Section 5.4 and Section 5.5. The gelatine filter dissolves on the surface of the agar plate.

5.4   Incubation

Incubate the plates as indicated in Section 1.4.5.

5.5   Reading and interpretation of results

Count all colonies and express results as cfu per m^3 (or cfu per volume sampled). Identify colonies as necessary.

6   Passive sampling for environmental microorganisms

6.1   Room settle plates and work area session plates for enumerating aerobic bacteria, moulds and yeasts

6.1.1   Materials

Settle plates are generally 90mm plates, preferably containing at least 20ml of sterile agar medium, and formulated to resist dehydration in isolators, cabinets or workstations.

Settle plates should be exposed for a maximum of four hours. If sessions are longer than four hours, a second set of plates should be exposed. Best practice is to record the length of actual exposure. The performance of agar plates is likely to be affected by desiccation, for example a water loss exceeding 20% of the original wet agar weight. This can lead to an underestimate of the number of organisms and needs to be considered when interpreting results. Best practice would be to establish the time taken for a weight loss of a maximum of 15% of the wet agar in the specific environment in which the plate is exposed.

If using plates with locking lids; after use, ensure the mechanism is closed correctly. This may be performed outside the critical work zone.

Note: The packaging of plates or swabs that are processed through a gaseous biodecontamination cycle into a critical work zone should be made from a material shown to be impermeable to the gassing agent.

6.1.2 Technique

At least three successful methods of exposure have been employed (see Figure B1.2).

Figure B1.2
Techniques of settle plate exposure

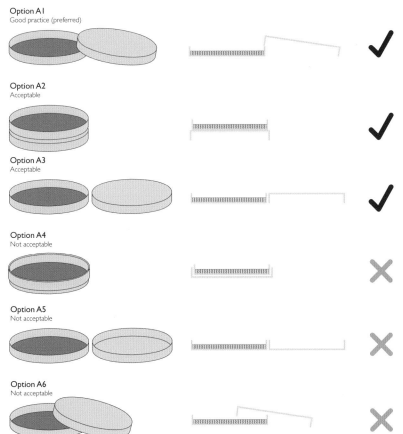

Option A1
Good practice (preferred)

Option A2
Acceptable

Option A3
Acceptable

Option A4
Not acceptable

Option A5
Not acceptable

Option A6
Not acceptable

Consideration of the individual circumstances is necessary, but in general terms, option A1 is best practice, options A2 and A3 are acceptable, and options A4, A5 and A6 are unacceptable.

At the end of the exposure period, replace the lid and remove the plate to a suitable area to secure the lid and place the plate in the original bag or suitable packaging.

6.1.3 Incubation

Incubate the plates, inverted, as indicated in Section 1.4.5.

6.1.4 Reading and interpretation of results

Count all individual colonies on each plate and express results as cfu per plate. Where cfus are merged, a sensible attempt to establish the number of colonies should be made. Agar that appears to be desiccated should be noted in the report as a possible indication of under reporting the true growth.

6.1.5 Too numerous to count (TNTC)

A common definition for TNTC is 200 or more cfu on a typical 90mm settle plate.

Identify colonies as appropriate, utilising visual macroscopic morphology in the first instance, followed by microscopy, staining and other biochemical tests. Refer to Figure B1.1.

6.2 Contact plates or strips/slides for surface sampling and environmental monitoring

If surfaces are not flat or accessible, e.g. corners, curved surfaces, irregular items and crevices, swab sampling should be used – see Section 6.3.

When contact plates or strips/slides are used for surface sampling, a validated procedure should be used to ensure adequate contact and dwell time, avoiding obscured or non-contact areas, e.g. trapped air bubbles. After application, excess culture medium transferred to the surface being sampled should be removed.

Contact plates or strips/slides can be used to determine the bioburden on transferred items or on garments after use.

Note: The working tip of the fingers and thumbs and the left and right hand prints should be clearly identified.

Any trace of medium remaining on the surfaces, or fingers sampled by contact with agar, should be immediately removed by wiping. Secure plates and label with unit details and return to the laboratory for incubation.

6.4.3 Incubation
Incubate the plates, inverted, as indicated in Section 1.4.5.

6.4.4 Reading and interpretation of results
Count all the colonies on each glove print and express results as cfu per gloved hand. Identify colonies as necessary; colonies should coincide with, i.e. be associated with, the impression from the finger dabs.

Where cfus are merged, a sensible attempt to establish the number of colonies should be made. Agar that appears to be desiccated should be noted in the report as a possible indication of under reporting the true growth.

Where no finger indent is discernible on the plate, comment to this effect should be made on the report and consideration given to whether this represents a valid or void result.

If colonies are detected on the plates but are not co-located with the finger indents, comment to this effect should be made on the report and consideration given to whether this constitutes a finger dab failure or environmental stray contamination.

Identify colonies, as appropriate, either by automated technique (see Table B1.3) or by utilising visual macroscopic morphology in the first incidence followed by microscopy, staining and other biochemical tests. Refer to Figure B1.1.

Count all the colonies on each glove print and express results as cfu per gloved hand. Identify colonies as necessary; colonies should coincide with the impression from the finger dabs.

7 Tap water sampling

Tap water is likely to contain low levels of disinfectant, for example chlorine, which can inhibit the growth of microorganisms and therefore any disinfectant should be inactivated or removed. Once inactivated, microorganisms may multiply if water is left to stand in the sampling container and therefore on-site testing, or transport to the laboratory within four hours, or refrigeration for up to 24 hours is recommended.

7.1.1 Materials

Sterile sampling containers with sodium thiosulphate (a neutralising agent for chlorine) are available for taking tap water samples.

A number of agars have been used for testing water. R2A has been recommended for potable water (BD 2009). For on-site testing, filter cassettes are available which use liquid media such as TSB or R2B (Atlas 2010).

7.1.2 Technique

Run the tap for the specified time before sampling, or sample immediately into a sterile container. If sodium thiosulphate is present in the sample container, it should be filled to the correct mark and either refrigerated or dispatched immediately to the laboratory.

If the water is to be tested immediately, pass 1ml through a field monitor (a type of microbial filter incorporating an absorbent pad for broth), followed by 10ml of Tryptone Soya Broth (TSB). Alternatively, wash the sample through with 10ml sterile water and then add 1ml of R2B medium to the pad. If the sample is sent to a laboratory, 1ml should be filtered through a 47mm 0.45µ cellulose nitrate sterile filter, washed with 10ml sterile water and the filter removed aseptically and transferred to a sterile R2A agar plate. Ensure that no air bubbles are trapped between the membrane filter and the medium. 'Rolling' the membrane filter onto the medium minimises the likelihood of air bubbles becoming trapped.

7.1.3 Incubation

A liquid medium in a field monitor should be incubated, inverted, for 3-5 days, as appropriate, at 25°C. Typically, agar with an attached membrane is incubated, inverted, for 5-7 days at 25°C.

7.1.4 Reading and interpretation of results

Count all colonies and express results as cfu per ml.

7.1.5 Too numerous to count (TNTC)

TNTC can be considered to be 100 or more cfu on a typical filter.

Identify colonies, as appropriate, either by utilising automated technique (see Table B1.3) or by visual macroscopic morphology in the first instance followed by microscopy, staining and other biochemical tests. Refer to Figure B1.1.

Identify colonies, as necessary, to at least genus level. The presence of Gram-negative microorganisms or other objectionable organisms should trigger an investigation.

8   Monitoring of material transfer procedures

All items transferred into a biodecontamination (gassing) isolator should be cleaned to remove dirt and grease just before the cycle. There is no requirement for routine monitoring of this cleaning process.

However, if a traditional isolator or unidirectional air flow cabinet is used, a sanitisation procedure should be carried out when transferring items into a higher grade area. The process is usually carried out using a spray-wipe process. As the technique is manual and dependent on individual operator skills, it is difficult to validate. Regular monitoring of each operator's technique is recommended either by surface sampling as described in Section 6.2 and/or 6.3 or bioburden testing (Hiom et al 2004). Bioburden testing is preferred as it tests all the surfaces, including difficult to clean areas such as inside folds, creases and crevices. An inactivator may be considered if a non-volatile disinfectant or sporicide has been used. The test should be carried out as follows:

8.1.1   Materials

- Sterile TSB or settle plates
- Sterile bag or sterile container
- Sterile wetting agent – 0.1% peptone and 0.1% Tween; sterile water; sterile quarter strength Ringers solution or sterile inactivator solution.

8.1.2   Technique

Place items for testing in a sterile bag, then seal and send to a microbiology laboratory for testing. At the laboratory, 100ml of wetting agent should be added to the bag and the contents agitated for two minutes. Withdraw 50ml and filter it through a 47mm 0.45μm mixed cellulose esters, sterile filter. If a filter with pad (field monitor) is used, moisten the pad with TSB. If there is no pad, aseptically remove the filter and layer it onto an agar plate.

Ensure that no air bubbles are trapped between the membrane filter and the medium. 'Rolling' the membrane filter onto the medium minimises the likelihood of air bubbles becoming trapped.

Contact plating of the items and/or the use of swabs can be considered as alternative methods, but have reduced sensitivity and recovery.

8.1.3 Incubation

Incubate the field monitor, inverted, for 5 days at 25°C. Incubate agar plates, inverted, as indicated in Section 1.4.5.

8.1.4 Reading and interpretation of results

Count all colonies and express results as cfu per number of items and compare 'before and after' results.

Note: Remember to take dilution factors into consideration and to calculate the result accordingly.

Identify colonies, as necessary, to at least genus level. The presence of microorganisms after the process should trigger an investigation.

9 Process validation by media fill

The process to be validated should be clearly identified (see Part B – 2.1). The starting materials should be substituted with sterile TSB in a similar container and closure system.

Note: Gamma irradiated TSB is available commercially as a powder for reconstitution for process validation tests. If this is not possible, microbiologically inert solutions may be permitted provided the strength of broth in the final container is proven to support growth. Double- or triple-strength TSB may be used provided the pH is carefully controlled. This, together with other strengths in a variety of packs, is available from commercial suppliers. The final concentration of the growth medium should equate to single strength +/- 10%.

9.1.1 Materials

TSB in appropriate containers.

9.1.2 Technique

The components in the process that have been substituted with broth, or a microbiologically inert substance, need to be identified. The operator(s) should follow the usual method, as described in the SOP, including the usual environmental monitoring techniques, in order to prepare the simulated product. Label the final product containers to clearly identify them as a process simulation product only. Send all intact media containers to the microbiology laboratory for incubation and examination.

9.1.3 Incubation

Incubate the medium (simulated product) for seven days at 20-25°C and examine for signs of growth. Gently agitate the container to ensure all surfaces are washed with medium and incubate for a further seven days at 30-35°C.

9.1.4 Reading and interpretation of results

The process validation is deemed to be satisfactory if, after the initial 14 days' incubation, the broth remains clear and, subsequently, the inoculated challenge exhibits growth. Any container exhibiting growth should be streaked out and the colonies identified, preferably to species level.

Media fertility is assured by inoculating the medium using 10-100cfu of test strains of organisms given in the current *British Pharmacopoeia*. The medium should be incubated with growth apparent after three days at 30-35°C in the case of bacteria and five days at 20-25°C in the case of fungi.

If the broth remains clear after challenging with a microorganism, a second challenge using the same organism is permitted. If this fails to grow, an out-of-specification investigation should be carried out to identify the reason. A reduction in pH is a sign of media degradation and could lead to poor growth.

Note: A failure in the sessional settle plates or finger dabs represents a process validation failure.

10 End of session media fill

End of session (EOS) media fills should evaluate all types of aseptic manipulations carried out in a workstation on a cyclic basis. Similarly all operators should be included on a rolling basis. Typically an end-of-session test mimics a preparation that has been carried out in a workstation using broth. EOS media fills may not be appropriate for radiopharmacy preparation as it is not possible to fully mimic the elution of a generator.

It is possible to transfer remnants of a container into broth or transfer broth into an in-process container, however, there should be no antimicrobial ingredients that will inhibit microorganism growth. The final concentration of the growth medium should equate to single strength broth +/- 10%. It is usual to produce a single final container for incubation, however, all intact media containers should be sent to a laboratory for incubation and examination.

Note: An EOS media fill is not equivalent to a sterility test because anaerobic organisms such as *Clostridia* will not grow in TSB, and it does not test the actual product.

10.1.1 Materials
Sterile TSB.

10.1.2 Technique
The manipulations should be carried out using the normal aseptic technique employed. Label the final product containers to clearly identify them as an end-of-session media fill. Send all intact media containers to a laboratory for incubation and examination.

10.1.3 Incubation
As described for process validation by media fill in Section 9.

10.1.4 Reading and interpretation of results
As described for process validation by media fill in Section 9.

11 Monitoring of disinfectant solutions

Surface cleaning is an important aspect of maintaining a clean room in a suitable condition for aseptic preparation (Rutala and Weber 2008).

Mops can be used to clean surfaces such as ceilings, walls and floors and there are a variety of liquid agents available to assist. These agents include non-ionic surfactants for removing chemical residues, disinfectants for killing vegetative microorganisms and sporicidal agents for killing all microorganisms.

It is important that the cleaning regime does not add to the bioburden and, therefore, testing of disinfectant solutions may be required. Pre-impregnated, sterile, cleaning systems are available and monitoring of these is not formally required. If, however, the disinfectants are prepared from concentrates and water, they should be tested before and after use.

11.1.1 Materials
- Sterile water
- Sterile inactivator solution with peptone
- Sterile TSB.

11.1.2 Technique

Transfer 1ml of the disinfectant solution into a 10ml syringe and filter through a 47mm 0.45μ mixed cellulose esters, sterile filter. Draw 50ml of sterile water into the syringe and pass through the filter. Draw 10ml of inactivator solution, validated for the disinfectant, into the syringe and pass through the filter. If a filter with a pad (field monitor) is used, moisten the pad with TSB. If there is no pad, aseptically remove the filter and layer onto an agar plate.

Ensure that no air bubbles are trapped between the membrane filter and the medium. 'Rolling' the membrane filter onto the medium minimises the likelihood of air bubbles becoming trapped.

11.1.3 Incubation

Incubate the field monitor, inverted, for 5-7 days at 25°C. Incubate agar plates, inverted, as indicated in Section 1.4.5.

11.1.4 Reading and interpretation of results

Count all colonies and express results as cfu per ml and compare 'before and after' results.

Identify colonies, as necessary, to at least genus level. The presence of microorganisms before the process should trigger an investigation. Identification to species level will assist when attempting to identify likely sources of organisms recovered in routine monitoring, especially contact plate results.

12   Interpretation of microbiology reports

The correct interpretation of microbiology reports, and appropriate handling of the data they contain, is of considerable importance in the correct management of controlled environments and aseptic processing. The data should be processed in a manner that ensures senior staff and key personnel are aware of critical parameters relating to the reports and are aware of their significance.

The following areas should be covered by the reporting system:

1. Data presentation

2. Alert levels and action limits

3. Reporting out-of-specification results

4. Trend analysis of results

5. Characteristics, significance and source of isolates.

12.1 Data presentation

Data should be presented in a clear and unambiguous way that enables the recipient to readily identify the premises, rooms, equipment, materials and personnel referred to in the report.

The report should contain at least the following:

- a unique reference number or code
- unit details and location
- laboratory details and location
- clear identification of all data points
- clear results for all data points
- date and temperature of incubation
- signature and date of person reading the results
- signature and date of the person releasing the results.

12.2 Alert levels and action limits

Appropriate alert levels and action limits should be set for all test criteria.

Alert levels should reflect situations where results are within limits, but are exceeding normal trends. They should be reviewed at least annually to determine whether they should be increased or decreased. If a result is outside the action limits, a review should be instigated as described in Section 12.4.

Action limits reflect situations where results are starting to indicate failure.

Clearly defined procedures should be in place to enable staff to respond effectively to the receipt of alert levels and action limit results. If a result is outside the action limits, an investigation should be instigated as described in Section 12.4.

12.3 Reporting out-of-specification results

When test results are outside specification, the laboratory should bring the result to the attention of the Accountable Pharmacist or deputy in the unit submitting the sample, as soon as possible. Results may be reported by telephone, electronically or fax. The laboratory should have a system to record who received the result and when. Advice on the likely source of the organism, and how to control the contamination, should be given by the testing laboratory. Particular importance should be placed on all organisms isolated during routine use in a biodecontamination isolator. Species identification will be required as a matter of urgency. Additional guidance is given in Section 13.

12.4 Guidance on actions to be taken when alert levels and action limits are exceeded

The following notes provide examples of actions which may be taken when levels are exceeded during room monitoring.

Alert level

- Check and review all environmental monitoring results and assess trends
- Identify microorganisms involved to genus level, and preferably to species level, if repeated alert levels are breached (MHRA 2015).

Action limit

- Review all environmental monitoring results and assess trends
- Identify microorganisms involved to genus level, and preferably to species level
- Record the need to take action in the Pharmaceutical Quality System (see Part A, Chapter 8)
- Carry out a risk assessment and consider the following options:
    - Additional monitoring
    - Additional cleaning
    - Observe operator technique
    - Counsel operators, consider re-training
    - Check work capacity and activity
    - Restrict shelf life of products (for example to less than 24 hours) (see Part B – 4)
    - Check for deviations to normal standard procedures
    - Halt aseptic preparation until the problem is resolved
    - Quarantine any product not issued
    - Check the workstation for malfunction.

12.5 Trend analysis of results

Trend analysis can be performed by any suitable method including:

- bar charts
- graphs
- cusum and shewhart plots
- exponential moving average.

An example of trending sessional settle plates or finger dabs is to determine the number of excursions in the last 40 results. In a unit used twice daily, Monday to Friday, this would represent a month's set of finger dabs or session plates. One failure would be represented as a 2.5% failure rate, two failures as 5% and three as 7.5%. Action should be taken at 2.5% to prevent an increase, such as additional cleaning based on the genus identification (see Section 13). If 5% is reached, the action taken at 2.5% may not have been effective and a more detailed investigation should be conducted and more extensive actions taken, e.g. by investigating operator technique. If 7.5% or more is reached, a full CAPA analysis should be carried out taking into account all the guidance given in Section 12.4, action limit.

Graphs and bar charts lend themselves to a manual process. Cusum and shewhart plots can be adopted but they are relatively complex and convoluted for environmental monitoring trends. A simpler technique, which lends itself to computerisation, is to determine whether the average is moving or not. Exponential moving averages (EMA) places slightly more emphasis on the current result and therefore less emphasis on historical data.

The following equation is used:-

$$EMA_n = result_n \times (2 / (t+1)) + EMA_{n-1} \times (1 - (2 / (t+1)))$$

where n is the current result and t is a fixed period or number of results to be included.

For a new aseptic unit, the first five results for a plate position are often used in qualification to determine whether the unit is in control and to determine the average result and standard deviation. An alert level is often set at this point. There is no standard way of calculating the alert level, however twice the average or the average + 2 standard deviations are often considered. For trending, the average is used for the first EMA_{n-1}. For a trend that is responsive to changes t = 5 could be used.

$$EMA_n = result_n \times 0.333 + EMA_{n-1} \times 0.667$$

Trends will often change direction if results fluctuate. For a more stable graph t = 13 is suggested.

$$EMA_n = result_n \times 0.143 + EMA_{n-1} \times 0.857$$

The graph will be less responsive to changes but may give a better idea whether the results are gradually getting higher or lower.

For long term trending it is suggested that t = 52 is used.

$$EMA_n = result_n \times 0.038 + EMA_{n-1} \times 0.962$$

At an annual review the value assigned to t should be reviewed and the alert levels for each plate position should be reassessed and changed if appropriate.

Note: If the alert level increases by a significant amount compared with that set for the previous period or begins to approach or exceeds the action limit, a CAPA investigation should be conducted as the room is not well-controlled.

13 Characteristics, significance and source of isolates

This guide has been produced to help in the interpretation of microbiological and environmental monitoring reports. Information on the common organism groups has been included, together with their likely source and treatment in a clean room setting.

13.1 Organism groups

The following section of this guide indicates the pathogenicity of some commonly-isolated microorganisms, together with the most likely sources of contamination.

It should be borne in mind that even those organisms that are of relatively low pathogenicity may be extremely hazardous under certain circumstances. It cannot be over stressed that the nature of any contamination found is at least as significant as the numbers of organisms detected.

As contaminants in aseptically-prepared medicines, these organisms may proliferate and cause a serious and possibly fatal infection, particularly when administered parenterally.

13.2 *Staphylococcus*

Gram-positive cocci (spheres). These form a large proportion of contaminants found in environmental monitoring samples.

The most notable member of this genus is *S. aureus*, which is a human pathogen. However, this organism is carried with no symptoms by a sizeable number of healthy adults. Some strains of *S. aureus* have become resistant to some antibiotics such as Methicillin and therefore have clinical significance. However, in aseptic preparation all *S. aureus* should be treated with equal concern.

Other species in this genus are generally harmless commensals found on human skin and in sputum, but have been implicated in opportunistic infections in immuno-compromised patients. These include:

- *S. epidermidis*
- *S. hominis*
- *S. saprophyticus*
- *S. capitis*.

These species are likely to be human in origin, as common sources include skin, hair, wounds, abscesses and clothing. However, the presence of these microorganisms in critical areas may not be due to the operator. Poor transfer disinfection may allow these microorganisms to be passed into clean areas. Dust, a high proportion of which is composed of shed human skin flakes, may also contain large numbers of *Staphylococcus*.

Identification of this genus is by colonial morphology and Gram staining. Differentiation between *S. aureus* and other species is by colony pigmentation, rapid identification techniques or the coagulase test.

This group of organisms is easily controlled using 70% alcohol solution and therefore, if present in a work area, may indicate poor cleaning techniques. On floors, a reduction in the numbers of microorganisms will occur by desiccation and the regular use of disinfectant agents.

13.3 *Micrococcus*

Gram-positive cocci: These are similar to commensal *Staphylococcus* species in terms of likely sources and clinical significance and are found frequently in environmental monitoring samples. The most common organisms in this group are *Micrococcus luteus*, and *Micrococcus lylae* and these frequently rank as the No 1 and No 2 most common organisms found in clean rooms.

This group of organisms is easily controlled using 70% alcohol solution and, therefore, if present in a work area could indicate poor cleaning or transfer techniques. On floors, a reduction in the numbers of these organisms will occur by the regular use of disinfectant agents.

13.4 *Streptococcus*

This group is rarely found in environmental monitoring samples, but common sources include throat infections, respiratory tract, wounds and abscesses. If the organism is introduced into the blood stream the consequences can be clinically significant for example, pneumonia.

This group of organisms is easily controlled using 70% alcohol solution and, therefore, if present in a work area could indicate poor handling and cleaning techniques. On floors, a reduction in the numbers of these organisms will occur by the regular use of disinfectant agents.

13.5 *Bacillus*

Large genus of spore-forming aerobic Gram-positive rods. The main pathogen in this group is *B. anthracis* (the causative agent of anthrax) which is highly unlikely to appear in environmental monitoring samples. Other species that may cause problems (bacteraemia, meningitis, endocarditis, etc.) in immuno-compromised patients include:

- *B. cereus*
- *B. sphaericus*
- *B. subtilis*.

Bacillus species may be saprophytes, commensals or pathogens; they may be isolated from personnel, soil, water, vegetation and foodstuffs. Their spores are formed as a response to unfavourable conditions and are ubiquitous in the environment. These spores are extremely resistant to desiccation, heat and many common disinfectants, and some are resistant to physical removal because they exude adhesive-like substances, e.g. *B. cereus*.

The presence of *Bacillus* species in environmental monitoring samples may be indicative of inadequate cleaning/disinfection or poor transfer disinfection. Common sources include dust, air (especially from draughts), cardboard, paper, water, mops and clothing.

This group of organisms are not easily controlled. *Bacilli* sporulate on exposure to air and are not killed by the routine disinfectants used in clean rooms. The simple act of cleaning can remove low numbers. Sporicidal agents such as hypochlorite, hypochlorous acid, hydrogen peroxide or peracetic acid have been developed for use to assist in removing these organisms and prevent them entering work areas.

13.6 Unidentified Gram-positive rods

Gram-positive rods not showing the presence of spores characteristic of *Bacillus* species: These may be *Bacillus* species that have not produced spores, or one of the species described here. Spores may not be formed in *Bacillus* cultures that have favourable growth conditions or have lost the ability to sporulate due to environmental conditions.

Pathogens in this group include:

- *Listeria monocytogenes*
- *Corynebacterium diphtheriae.*

Neither of these species is likely to be found in environmental monitoring samples. Most of the other organisms in this group are generally harmless commensals of human origin, or found in soil and plants. Diptheroids, such as the above, are commonly found on the skin.

This group of organisms is easily controlled using routine disinfectant agents.

13.7 *Pseudomonads*

Large group of Gram-negative rods: They are highly adaptable organisms with very low nutrient requirements and a high innate resistance to many common disinfectants and antibiotics. Widely distributed in nature as saprophytes, commensals and pathogens for humans, plants, animals and insects, these species are commonly found in water samples.

A number of species are opportunistic pathogens i.e. unlikely to cause disease in healthy adults, but may do so in patients whose immune system is compromised in some way, and may be particularly debilitating in respiratory and ophthalmic infections. This group includes:

- *Pseudomonas aeruginosa*
- *P. fluorescens*
- *P. stutzeri*
- *Burkholderia cepacia* (formally named *P. cepacia*)
- *Stenotropomonas maltophilia* (formally named *P. maltophilia*)
- *Sphingomonas paucimobilis* (formally named *P. paucimobilis*).

P. aeruginosa is the most prominent member of the above group, and is found as a saprophyte in warm, moist environments including hot and cold water systems, sinks, drains and even disinfectant solutions if not correctly prepared and used.

Under certain conditions, it and other members of this genus may form a protective film (known as a biofilm) which can help the organism survive attack by disinfectants in pipe work, water tanks etc. For this reason the presence of *Pseudomonas* in the aseptic unit hand-wash water should be acted upon and either flushed down the drain, or the supply water chemically treated. A re-test should confirm the organism has been removed.

All members of the genus are killed easily by heat and so present little challenge to autoclaving. However, due to the nature of their cell walls (as with other Gram-negative organisms) and an ability to exude a slime coating, they may lead to increased endotoxin (pyrogen) levels. They are also very susceptible to desiccation and, hence, keeping surfaces and equipment as clean and dry as possible will help to reduce the incidence of *Pseudomonas* contamination.

Identification of the genus is by colonial morphology and Gram staining, combined with simple biochemical tests (oxidase and catalase tests). More detailed identification to species level may require subculture onto selective media (and looking for production of certain pigments), or the use of API or similar biochemical test systems.

Biofilms are not easy to control without some form of abrasion and treating areas before they become established is recommended (DH 2012).

It is recommended that all taps associated with an aseptic suite are run for at least 2 minutes before use and sinks are disinfected daily. Regular monitoring of the sink should be carried out (see Part A – 7.1.22 and Part A 11.9).

Bacteria within biofilms may be up to 1,000 times more resistant to antimicrobials than are the same bacteria in suspension. Chlorine based disinfectants including chloramines may effectively inactivate biofilm bacteria (Rutala and Weber 2008). *Burkholderia cepacia* has been shown to be particularly problematic as it can form biofilms on stainless steel surfaces and is difficult to remove due to its adhesion to the metal (Nörnberg et al 2011). If present in an isolator, it may require repeated sanitisation to fully eliminate the contamination.

13.8   Enterobacteria

Gram-negative bacilli or cocci bacilli bacteria are differentiated from *Pseudomonads* by their negative response to the oxidase test. This group includes the following genera (though not exclusively):

- *Acinetobacter spp*
- *Enterobacter spp*
- *Escherichia spp (e.g. E. coli)*
- *Klebsiella spp*
- *Proteus spp*
- *Salmonella spp*
- *Serratia spp*
- *Shigella spp.*

These organisms are generally (although by no means all) found in the intestinal tract of humans and animals, and hence can also be found in faecal matter and sewage. Some are primary pathogens (causing a range of intestinal infections, bacteraemia and endotoxin shock), although many are commensals and saprophytes. Therefore, precise identification using biochemical testing is important should organisms from this group be isolated.

Acinetobacter spp. are aerobic 'rod-shaped', non-motile Gram-negative cocci bacilli that look similar to *haemophilus influenzae* on Gram stain. Commonly present in soil and water as free-living saprophytes. There are many species; all can cause human disease, as opportunistic pathogens.

Certain *Acinetobacter spp.*, chiefly *A. johnsonii, A. lwoffii* and *A. radioresistens*, are part of the bacterial flora of the skin. *A. baumannii* is a multi-resistant organism sensitive to relatively few antibiotics.

As with *Pseudomonas* species, the presence of enterobacteria may lead to elevated endotoxin levels.

Sporicidal agents such as hypochlorite, hypochlorous acid, hydrogen peroxide or peracetic acid are recommended to assist in removing these organisms and prevent them entering work areas.

13.9   Unidentified Gram-negative rods

These organisms are most likely to be found in water samples. Further identification may be difficult, although this will be of importance in aseptic units where their presence is undesirable, however the laboratory should confirm that the organism is truly Gram-negative – see Section 3.1.3, before action is taken as described for *Pseudomonas* in Section 13.7.

This group of organisms is easily controlled using routine disinfectant agents.

13.10 Moulds

Spore-producing saprophytic fungi ubiquitous in normal environments, particularly favouring cooler, damp conditions: They have low-nutrient requirements and can thrive on walls and ceilings. They are often released into the atmosphere, since they are associated with building work. Mould spores are often found in soil, garden mulch, dust and untreated cardboard and paper. A number of species are opportunistic pathogens. Common contaminants in clean room environments include:

- *Cladosporium spp*
- *Aspergillus spp*
- *Penicillium spp*
- *Fusarium spp.*

The occasional colony of mould isolated in clean rooms may not be a major cause for concern, but all moulds should be considered as 'objectionable' organisms and action taken accordingly.

Moulds found in critical environments are generally indicative of inadequate cleaning or poor transfer disinfection.

Many common disinfectants have limited activity against moulds and hence they are very difficult to eradicate completely once they have obtained a foothold in the fabric of buildings. Hypochlorite solutions are quite effective and give a rapid kill.

13.11 Yeasts

Fungi found as part of commensal flora on skin: Common sources include personnel and foodstuffs. Opportunistic pathogens include:

- *Candida albicans*
- *Candida glabrata*
- *Cryptococcus neoformans.*

This group of organisms is easily controlled using routine disinfectant agents.

13.12 Actinomycetes/Streptomyces

The phrase 'Actinomycetes' refers to a group of Gram-positive filamentous bacteria including the genera *Streptomyces*, *Nocardia* and *Actinomyces*.

Actinomyces are commensal microorganisms found in the mouth and intestine. They are unlikely to be found in routine environmental monitoring.

Nocardia are soil and dust saprophytes. They may occasionally cause a chronic infection known as mycetoma.

Streptomyces are soil and dust saprophytes that form spores similar to those produced by moulds. They are often in environmental monitoring samples, particularly from relatively dirty areas. They rarely cause mycetoma, except in immuno-compromised patients.

Dermatophytes are the most widely distributed fungal infection of humans and *Trichophyton rubrum* is the most common cause of tinea infections, e.g. ringworm, athlete's foot, jock itch and similar complaints. Almost certain to be present in changing rooms, but rarely detected due to a slow growth profile.

Sporicidal agents such as hypochlorite, hypochlorous acid, hydrogen peroxide or peracetic acid are recommended to assist in removing these organisms and to prevent them entering work areas.

14 Suitable media formulae

14.1 Media formulations (from BP/USP 2016)

Tryptone Soya Broth	g/ l
Pancreatic digest of casein (Tryptone)	17.0
Papaic digest of Soya bean meal	3.0
Sodium chloride	5.0
Dipotassium hydrogen phosphate	2.5
Dextrose monohydrate	2.5
Water	1000.0ml
pH 7.3 ± 0.2	

Tryptone Soya Agar	g/ l
Pancreatic digest of casein (Tryptone)	15.0
Soya peptone	5.0
Sodium chloride	5.0
Agar	15.0
Water	1000.0ml
pH 7.3 ± 0.2	

Sabouraud Dextrose Agar	g/ l
Mycological peptone	10.0
Dextrose monohydrate	40.0
Agar	15.0
Water	1000.0ml
pH 5.6 ± 0.2	

Tryptone Soya Agar with inactivators	g/ l
Pancreatic digest of casein (Tryptone)	15.0
Soya peptone	5.0
Sodium chloride	5.0
Lecithin	0.7
Tween 80	5.0
Sodium thiosulphate	0.5
Histidine	1.0
Agar	15.0
Water	1000.0ml
pH 7.3 ± 0.2	

Sabouraud Dextrose Agar with inactivators	g/ l
Mycological peptone	10.0
Dextrose monohydrate	40.0
Lecithin	0.7
Tween 80	5.0
Sodium thiosulphate	0.5
Histidine	1.0
Agar	15.0
Water	1000.0ml
pH 5.6 ± 0.2	

14.2 Non-Pharmacopoeial formulations

Inactivator solution	g/ l
Lecithin	20
Tween 80	30
Sodium thiosulphate	10
Water	1000.0ml
pH at 25 °C 7.0 ± 0.2	

Inactivator solution with peptone	g/ l
Lecithin	20
Tween 80	30
Sodium thiosulphate	10
Peptone	100
Water	1000.0ml
pH at 25 °C 7.0 ± 0.2	

Tryptone Soya Agar with glucose	g/ l
Pancreatic digest of casein	15
Enzymatic digest of soya bean	5
Sodium Chloride	5
Agar	15
Glucose	10
Water	1000.0ml
pH at 25 °C 7.0 ± 0.2	

References

Atlas RM (2010). *Handbook of Microbiological Media.* 4th edn. London: CRC Press. p1472.

Barnett HL, Hunter B (1987). *Illustrated Genera of Fungi.* 4th edn. London: Macmillan.

Barrow GI, Feltham RKA eds (2003). *Cowan and Steel's Manual for the Identification of Medical Bacteria.* 3rd edn. Cambridge: Cambridge University Press.

Becton, Dickinson and Company (BD) (2009). *Difco™ & BBL™ Manual.* 2nd edn. Maryland: Sparks. pp461-462.

Bridson E (2002). *The Oxoid Vade-Mecum of Microbiology.* Darby, PA: DIANE Publishing Company.

British Pharmacopoeia Commission Secretariat. *British Pharmacopoeia.* Current edn. London: The Stationery Office.

Department of Health (DH) (2012). *Water sources and potential Pseudomonas aeruginosa contamination of taps and water systems.* Leeds: DH. Paragraphs 16-17.

European Commission (2015). *The rules governing medicinal products in the European Community. Vol IV. Good Manufacturing Practice for medicinal products.* Available at: **http://ec.europa.eu/health/documents/eudralex/vol-4/index_en.htm** (accessed 26 February 2016).

Hayes JE, Hunt PB (2003). *Investigation into the optimum technique for surface sampling in cleanroom and controlled environments. Poster presentation at QC Symposium, October 2003.*

Hiom SJ et al (2004). Development and validation of a method to assess alcohol transfer disinfection procedures. *Pharm J* 272: 611.

Medicines and Healthcare products Regulatory Agency (MHRA) (2015). *Questions and Answers for Specials Manufacturers.* London: MHRA. Available at: **https://www.gov.uk/government/publications/guidance-for-specials-manufacturers** (accessed 19 February 2016).

Nörnberg MFBL et al (2011). A psychrotrophic Burkholderia cepacia strain isolated from refrigerated raw milk showing proteolytic activity and adhesion to stainless steel. *J Dairy Res* 78(3): 257-62.

Rhodes J et al (2016). The use of tryptone soya agar with 1% glucose for the environmental monitoring of pharmacy aseptic units. *The European Journal of Parenteral and Pharmaceutical Sciences* 21(2): 50-55.

Rutala WA, Weber DJ (2008). *Guideline for Disinfection and Sterilization in Healthcare Facilities.* Healthcare Infection Control Practices Advisory Committee. Atlanta: Centers for Disease Control and Prevention.

Sutton SVW (2012). What is an 'objectionable organism'? *American Pharmaceutical Review* 15(6). Available at: **http://www.americanpharmaceuticalreview.com/Featured-Articles/122201-What-is-an- Objectionable-Organism-Objectionable-Organisms-The-Shifting-Perspective/** (accessed 18 July 2016).

PART B – 2.1: MICROBIOLOGICAL VALIDATION OF THE PROCESS

Objective

To demonstrate that the procedures used during aseptic preparation, and the staff undertaking aseptic processes, are capable of maintaining the sterility of the product.

Principles

1   A process simulation is a validation procedure that challenges not only the method but the operator and the facilities. The test is intended to simulate routine aseptic operations but uses microbiological media to produce broth-filled units that can then be tested for contamination (PHSS1993). Sessional settle plates should be exposed, and finger dabs performed, as part of the process validation.

2   Procedures and facilities will be different depending on the type of product being prepared. Each operation should be analysed and a sequence devised that reflects the most complex practice for that product type, for example parenteral nutrition (PN) compounded from individual constituents is more complex than additions made to a standard PN bag. All product types prepared in the unit should be simulated e.g. filling of elastomeric devices, intrathecals prepared using non-luer equipment, PN prepared using auto compounders. Different tests are likely to be required to simulate different types of product with varying complexity.

Note: It is not possible to fully simulate the elution of a ^{99m}Tc generator using broth, as it is important to assure the sterility of the generator throughout its use. Sterility testing of finished product is required to provide assurance that the process is capable of maintaining the sterility of the product (see Part A, Chapter 11).

3   It may be that the Universal Operator Broth Transfer Validation Test (see Part B – 2.2) simulates many of the preparation processes within the unit. The number and type of manipulations should, however, be checked to ensure it reflects the worst case situation.

4   The number of units filled should reflect the maximum number of that type of product prepared in a single session.

5   Process validation, using broth to simulate the aseptic procedure, should be performed three times initially and subsequently at least on a six-monthly basis. A programme using different operators and all appropriate workstations should be prepared. The programme should be constructed so that validations are carried out throughout the year to take account of possible seasonal fluctuations such as background bioburdens or staffing levels. Process validation can form part of the periodic review of aseptic technique to supplement operator validation tests (see Part A – 11.3.5). New processes, or changes to existing processes, including the scale of the activity, should be assessed to ensure that previous process validations remain valid (MHRA 2015).

6   Tryptone soya broth would normally be used for these studies. This may be of double- and occasional triple-strength to allow for dilution during the test. The broth used should be assessed for fertility after use, as described in Part B – 1.

7   Broth-filled units should be incubated at the designated temperature for 14 days (see Part B – 1). If the final container is part filled, all surfaces should be in contact with the broth at some time during incubation. A pass result requires no growth in all containers, sessional settle plates and finger dabs following incubation.

8   There should be a thorough investigation as part of the corrective and/or preventative action (CAPA) process (see Part A, Chapter 8) following any genuine positive results. This should focus initially on whether the facilities, processes or operator practices are the likely cause of the failure. A review of all monitoring and test data since the previous process validation test should be carried out and implications for the products prepared considered and recorded. Revalidation of the process will be required.

References

Pharmaceutical and Healthcare Sciences Society (PHSS) (1993). *The Use of Process Simulation Tests in the Evaluation of Processes for the Manufacture of Sterile Products: Technical Monograph no 4.* Swindon: PHSS.

Medicines and Healthcare products Regulatory Agency (MHRA) (2015). *Questions and Answers for Specials Manufacturers.* London: MHRA. Available at: **https://www.gov.uk/government/publications/guidance-for-specials-manufacturers** (accessed 19 February 2016).

PART B – 2.2: MICROBIOLOGICAL VALIDATION OF THE OPERATOR

Objective

To demonstrate that the aseptic technique of the operator undertaking the aseptic process is capable of maintaining the sterility of the product.

Principles

1   All aseptic manipulations can be broken down into a number of key techniques:

- withdrawing solution from an infusion bag
- withdrawing solution from a vial
- withdrawing solution from an ampoule
- addition of solution to an infusion bag
- addition of solution to a vial.

2   The operator validation encompasses both regular aseptic manipulations and transfer sanitisation. All operators need to demonstrate competency in these techniques in order that they may prepare dosage units safely. To reduce variables, best practice is that the operator should undertake the transfer sanitisation of the components and broth to be used. This has the advantage of providing some assurance of the operator's transfer sanitisation technique. Sessional settle plates should be exposed and finger dabs performed as part of the validation.

3   Staff should initially carry out a minimum of three successful consecutive operator validation tests as part of their training programme. At least one of the initial tests should be supervised (normally this would be the first). Following this initial validation, a continuing programme of staff validation (at least six-monthly) should be established for all staff who use the aseptic unit. Validations should be rotated through differing types of clean air devices (pharmaceutical isolators and unidirectional air flow cabinets) used by the operator.

4   In the event of broth growth failure, the operator should be temporarily suspended, from aseptic preparation whilst a thorough investigation, as part of the CAPA process (see Part A, Chapter 8), is completed. Actions taken following the investigation should be made on a risk assessment basis. For a genuine broth failure this should include the operator undertaking a revalidation of three successful consecutive operator validation tests. Sessional settle plate or finger dab failures need not necessarily require suspension from preparation duties but should initiate an investigation of transfer and aseptic techniques and require a single successful operator validation retest as a minimum.

Universal Operator Broth Transfer Validation Test (UOBTV Test)

This is a standard assessment for operators prior to undertaking aseptic preparation activities and for routine operator revalidation. The test procedure is designed to emulate the manipulations described here which are used routinely in pharmacy aseptic preparation. Details of this test can be found on the NHS Pharmaceutical Aseptic Services Group website (**www.pasg.nhs.uk**).

Note: Radiopharmacies may find this test does not reflect their usual processes and a purpose-designed test may be more appropriate.

All operators should perform the required number of transfers in the specified order, to and from the required containers, using procedures and equipment with which they are familiar and that are currently in use in the unit in which they are working. For units wishing to consider accepting a UOBTV test for an operator transferring from another unit, the Accountable Pharmacist should consider and make a judgement as to the extent to which this might be transferable. Factors to be considered would include knowledge of the processes within the unit in which the UOBTV test was undertaken (to ensure results are transferable), evidence of the test results, and the experience of the operator. Use of this test also allows for benchmarking comparisons between aseptic units and data analysis on a wider basis.

The UOBTV test is not intended to replace the process-specific validation tests (see Part B – 2.1) which are applicable to the types of product prepared in a particular unit.

PART B – 2.3: PRODUCT VALIDATION

Objective

To confirm that the processes used will consistently produce a product that is suitable for the patient, containing the correct constituents at a concentration that is within acceptable limits, and that the chemical and microbiological integrity of the product can be assured throughout its designated shelf life.

Principles

1   The stability of the product, up to and during the time of administration, (including during infusion via implanted reservoirs) should be proven and is a prerequisite for validation of the composition of the finished product.

2   The container of the finished product should be capable of maintaining its integrity, in respect of microbial and chemical contamination, up to the point of use.

It is important that containers are purchased to a recognised standard in order to maintain a consistent design and quality; all such containers should be CE-marked medical devices. It should be remembered that certain containers, e.g. disposable plastic syringes, are not designed for the prolonged storage of medicines and cannot be assumed to be suitable for this purpose. Tests to validate the integrity of these containers, and their ongoing compliance, should be used to assess the acceptability of the syringe package as a final container. Syringe closure integrity can be assessed by filling the various types and sizes of syringe with a sterile medium (Tryptone Soya Broth). The containers should then be stored under a variety of conditions that simulate the challenges of storage and transport. The media should be incubated at a temperature that promotes growth (see Part B – 1, section 9). The outside of the container may be positively challenged by immersing in a medium containing a microbial culture and noting any subsequent growth. Chemical tests which detect leakage may also be used. The standards set out in microbiological protocol for the integrity testing of syringes should be followed (PQAC 2013). The results of such tests are specific to the particular syringe/cap combinations (size, manufacturer, part number, sterilisation method etc.). All container/cap combinations should be demonstrated to prevent the ingress of microorganisms using microbiological or physical testing. Syringes used for long-term storage should also be shown to comply with the *British Pharmacopoeia (BP)* specification for plastic syringes at the end of the storage period (BP Commission Secretariat, current edition).

3   Documentation should include a recorded check that the correct ingredients and components have been used. Validation should confirm that this process is effective in producing products within specification and fit for purpose. Validation of the constituents of the product is achieved by carrying out a schedule of chemical or other appropriate analyses of the finished product and/or intermediate stage that focuses on the critical constituents.

4   Validation of the microbiological quality of the product is achieved by carrying out a schedule of microbiological analysis (sterility testing) of the finished product, or by using media simulations representative of the process. A matrix approach should be used but all product types and processes should be validated independently (see Part A, Chapter 11).

5   The results of traditional microbiological analysis of the product will only be known in retrospect. There are newer rapid microbiological techniques which may be useful for aseptically-prepared product testing. The microbiological analysis of the finished product should not be confused with the *BP* sterility test (BP Commission Secretariat, current edition), as the requirements for volume taken and the number of containers cannot generally be met. The ability to carry out a retest in the event of an invalidated test is also unlikely. Any growth should be thoroughly investigated and a full root cause analysis should be carried out. Comparison may be made between different aseptic units as part of an external quality control scheme, such as Pharmassure.

6   The number and frequency of samples to be analysed, both chemically and microbiologically, is at the discretion of the individual unit. However, there are minimum expectations in order to maintain a robust validation status, as required in Part A. Particular attention should be paid to new procedures, automated processes and any process involving a bulk stage.

7   The validation status of all processes should be reviewed on an annual, or minimum biennial, basis to include a review of all relevant data generated for a process (operator, process, end of session media fill data and sterility testing data). Any shortfall in information to assure on-going validation should be addressed with specific validation studies. The validation review should be documented and can be incorporated into a Product Quality Review for the product group.

References

British Pharmacopoeia Commission Secretariat. *British Pharmacopoeia.* Current edn. London: The Stationery Office.

NHS Pharmaceutical Quality Assurance Committee (PQAC) (2013). *Protocols for the Integrity Testing of Syringes.* 2nd edn. Microbiology Protocols Group and NHS Pharmaceutical Research and Development Group (R and D).

PART B – 2.4: VALIDATION OF TRAINING

Objective

To confirm that the training programme is fit for purpose and that all staff have achieved a satisfactory level of knowledge and competency for the duties they are required to undertake.

Key considerations

- Effective training is a critical part of the quality assurance of aseptic products. It is important that both the training programme and the impact on the trainee are effective
- The training programme should be fully documented and constructed in a fashion that enables outcomes to be stated in terms of competencies, which are measurable.

Validation process

Effectiveness of the training programme

1   The training programme should be validated by:

   (i)   auditing the content by comparison with the appropriate elements of Good Manufacturing Practice (GMP) (EC 2015) (or updated editions)

   (ii)   checking that all necessary elements of the practical aspects of aseptic processing are incorporated within the programme (see the references section for relevant source documents)

   (iii) ensuring that the documentation of training undertaken is comprehensive, including records of experience and competency

   (iv)   a review by an experienced trainer (not necessarily involved in the aseptic service) to ensure that all appropriate steps for effective training are incorporated and that adequate records are maintained.

2   The training programme may be validated by assessing competency data from trainees before training, after training and after further time intervals to ensure that the programme is effective.

Effectiveness of training the operator

Assessment should focus on qualitative and not quantitative aspects, e.g. demonstration of good aseptic technique rather than how fast the task can be accomplished.

Assessors should be able to make confident decisions on competence, based on evidence from a number of sources.

Primary methods of assessing the effectiveness of training staff are observation (may be called Directly Observed Procedures – DOP) and supported questioning. Other methods may be used to supplement these, including simulation and written questioning. They should be used where there is a lack of opportunity for the individual to demonstrate competence at work or if significant risk is associated with assessed tasks. Written questioning may also be used as a development tool, to confirm achievement of learning objectives, or as a precursor to work-based assessment.

Additionally, case-based discussions (CBD) may be of benefit, as described on the National School of Healthcare Science (NSHCS) website.

For senior staff, 360 degree feedback (may be called multi-source feedback – MSF) can be a useful technique to assess the level of competency (see NSHCS website).

NHS nationally recognised frameworks are available for demonstration of competency in pre- and in- process accuracy checking, and product approval in aseptics (ASAWG 2014).

NHS Technical Specialist Education and Training group (TSET) have developed an online professional development portal (**www.tpdportal.org.uk**) where individuals can develop a personal competency profile, upload evidence of competence and create an electronic training plan.

There is also a TSET Aseptic Processing program (accessed via **www.tset.org.uk**) which is an e-learning training package that encompasses the basic concepts of aseptic preparation and GMP. The programme provides online computer-based learning, with downloadable documents, assessments and certification of achievement.

References

European Commission (2015). *The rules governing medicinal products in the European Community. Vol IV. Good Manufacturing Practice for medicinal products.* Available at: ***http://ec.europa.eu/health/documents/eudralex/vol-4/index_en.htm*** (accessed 26 February 2016).

National School of Healthcare Science (NSHCS). *Case Based Discussion (CBD)* [online, video]. Available at: ***https://olat.nshcs.org.uk/article/cbd-video-guide*** (accessed 26 May 2016).

National School of Healthcare Science (NSHCS). *MSF Video Guide* [online]. Available at: ***https://olat.nshcs.org.uk/article/msf-video-guide*** (accessed 26 May 2016).

NHS Aseptic Services Accreditations Working Group (ASAWG) (2014). *Nationally Recognised Competency Framework for Pharmacists and Pharmacy Technicians: Product Approval (Release) in Aseptic Services under Section 10 Exemption.* Available at: ***www.nhspedc.nhs.uk/supports.htm*** (accessed 26 May 2016).

NHS Technical Specialist and Education Training group (TSET). Available at: ***www.tset.org.uk*** (accessed 26 May 2016).

QUALITY ASSURANCE OF ASEPTIC PREPARATION SERVICES:
STANDARDS HANDBOOK PART B

PART B – 2.5: VALIDATION OF CLEANING PROCESSES

Objective

To confirm that chemical, microbiological and other contaminants are removed or inactivated during cleaning processes.

Principles

Tests should be carried out to provide evidence that the cleaning agent will remove any soiling or contamination of the surface, item or equipment and leave the surface free from residues and microbial contamination.

Microbiological cleaning validation includes assessing activity of the disinfectant against local isolates of bacteria, bacterial spores and fungi, checking to ensure that all detergents and disinfectants are mutually compatible and that appropriate rinsing will produce a result that meets the cleanliness specification of the surface, item or equipment.

Chemical cleaning validation includes assessing the ability of the cleaning agent to remove or inactivate key or indicator substances, for example drug residues, disinfectants and surfactants.

Effective cleaning and sanitisation is an important part of operating an aseptic unit as described in Part A, Chapter 12. There are several different cleaning and sanitisation processes that should be detailed in procedures and require validation (see also Part A – 12.9).

The method for validation should be specific to the application i.e. what is being cleaned. It is not possible to validate cleaning or sanitisation unless there is an appropriate detectable challenge. However, it is not good practice to deliberately contaminate an operational clean room or items transferred into such a room. It may be useful to consider a 'worst case scenario' i.e. the selection of a target chemical entity that can be recovered and detected in very low concentrations, and/or be hard to remove from a surface. If the cleaning is effective for the worst case conditions, effectiveness can be assured for other materials. Ideally, this will be an item routinely used in the environment and should not require deliberate 'seeding', but the latter may be an option.

The locations selected for sampling should be based on knowledge of the use of the environment and should reflect the most likely sites for the recovery of contaminants.

Procedures

Floor cleaning

When a new or refurbished aseptic facility is being commissioned, this provides a good opportunity to validate floor cleaning, e.g. as part of the performance qualification (PQ) and process validation (PV).

If the unit is left free of dust and dirt but not microbiologically clean, a challenge to the floor cleaning agents, equipment and procedure can be established.

Contact plates with suitable inactivators should be used before treatment and after every stage of cleaning. It is recommended that a sterile, neutral or non-ionic detergent is used first, followed by the selected disinfectants, and finally a sporicidal agent. If the cleaning procedure incorporates a process to remove sporicidal residues, the testing with contact plates should be undertaken after this removal. Identification of organisms to genus level will assist with interpretation of the test results.

Ongoing validation can be achieved by reviewing contact plates, floor swabs and microorganism identification results. The review of microbiological data can be used to inform the process for defining the frequency of both cleaning activities and revalidation of the environment.

If cleaning solutions are prepared in the unit, the process should be validated as described in Part B – 1, Section 11.

Chemical removal

Chemical contaminants originate from a variety of sources and the techniques adopted for removal (cleaning) and testing methods will vary. Removal of chemical contamination from key surfaces may include disinfectant residues, antibiotics, cytotoxic drugs, monoclonal antibodies and other biological substances, etc. In some cases, sampling kits can be obtained from test laboratories.

a) Disinfectant removal

The repeated application of disinfectant substances can result in a build-up of organic and other substances that microorganisms can use for survival and reproduction. A review of wipe or swab test results compared with contact plate results can be an indirect indication of a problem if the number of organisms found on the wipe or swab is significantly higher than routine contact plate monitoring results.

Validating a process for disinfectant removal can be achieved using swabs or wipes wetted with sterile water, and the swabs or wipes then tested for total organic carbon (TOC).

Validating the process of neutralising oxidising sporicidal agents such as hydrogen peroxide or hyperchlorous acid may be undertaken using potassium iodide test papers.

b) Equipment cleaning

The equipment used in aseptic preparation should be free from chemicals to prevent cross contamination and subsequent contamination of product containers. Of particular concern are cytotoxic, antibiotic and potent biologically-derived medicines. Swabs are the sampling method of choice, as they can access hard-to-reach areas. However, care in selection is needed and the test laboratory should be able to advise on the nature of the swab material and the test methodology.

Aseptic transfer disinfection

Validation will require a 'before and after' methodology to demonstrate the effective removal of the bioburden. This can be achieved either by surface sampling or bioburden testing (Cockcroft et al 2001).

Note: it is important that there is a 'challenge' to the transfer process and this should be representative of the 'normal' micro flora of the objects being transferred. This would normally include spores.

Bioburden testing is generally preferred as it tests all the surfaces including difficult-to-clean areas such as inside folds, creases and crevices (Hiom et al 2004) and assesses the challenge to the aseptic transfer process.

Considerable variation in technique may be demonstrated by individual operators, even when following a defined procedure. Therefore an aseptic transfer validation, including observation, should be considered for new operators, or those returning after a prolonged break. Routine monitoring of competence can be included as part of operator validation (see Part B – 2.2).

Hand preparation

It is important that all staff entering an aseptic facility wash hands prior to entry (see Part A, Chapter 10). This is to remove dirt or other soiling, excess sebum or similar fatty residues, and minimise microbial carry-over.

A 'before and after' methodology for validation is recommended to demonstrate the effective removal of soiling and bioburden.

Note: Visual inspection can be usefully applied.

Validation procedures vary and may include:

- Use of contact plates
- Use of microbial swabbing methods
- Fluorescent dye techniques – This is a favoured method as it can clearly show effectiveness of cleaning of the whole hand
- Surfactant 'stripping' solutions.

Considerable variation in technique may be demonstrated by individual operators, even when following a defined procedure. Therefore hand preparation validation should be considered for new operators, or those returning after a prolonged break. Periodic or random monitoring of competence is also recommended.

References

Cockcroft MG et al (2001). Validation of liquid disinfection techniques for transfer of components into hospital pharmacy clean rooms. *Hospital Pharmacy* 8: 226-232.

Hiom SJ et al (2004). Development and validation of a method to assess alcohol transfer disinfection procedures. *Pharm J* 272: 611.

PART B – 2.5: VALIDATION OF CLEANING PROCESSES

PART B – 2.6: COMPUTERISED SYSTEM VALIDATION

Objective

To confirm that computer hardware and software (collectively termed a computerised system) perform to the standards required by EU GMP Annex 11 (EC 2015) and the principles of Good Automated Manufacturing Practice (GAMP) (ISPE 2008) delivering an output that meets the user requirements, is accurate and free of errors.

Validation of a computerised system

A holistic approach is required for validation of computerised and automated systems. The system is not just the software which produces the label, worksheet etc. but also the PC hardware running the software and any printers connected to that PC in addition to any network connecting the system to the wider hospital infrastructure. It is essential that all of these components work as expected otherwise the desired outcome (for example a clear, accurate, legible label to put on a product) cannot be achieved.

Key considerations

■ Where a computerised system replaces a manual operation, there should be no resultant decrease in product quality, process control or quality assurance. There should be no increase in the overall risk of the process.

■ Where a computerised system is part of a wider network, the validation of the system should take into account the effect of the network on the operation of the system, especially with respect to the resilience of the network and any potential for data loss. When changes to the network are made, consideration should be given as to the degree of revalidation required. Arrangements should be made to ensure that the Accountable Pharmacist is informed of any relevant problems with, or changes to, the network.

■ Wherever possible the support of the organisation's Information Technology (IT) department should be sought, with IT staff being seen as external contractors and a suitable written agreement put in place to ensure appropriate continuity of service. Depending on the complexity of the system and the level of support needed, this may take the form of a detailed Technical (Quality)

Agreement (see also Part B – 3), or a service level agreement detailing basic quality requirements. At the very least, responsibility for notifying key users of proposed changes to systems, software upgrades etc. before the change is made should be clear (with the emphasis on formal change control).

- A standardised approach to validating all computerised systems should be used and documented in a Validation Master Plan (VMP).
- The level of resource put into validating a system should be commensurate with the risk posed by system failure – e.g. a system which calculates stability of a parenteral nutrition solution carries a higher risk of failure than a system for printing delivery labels for ward boxes, and hence would need a much greater level of validation effort.
- If the computerised system is replacing a manual process, operation of the two systems in parallel for an appropriate period with comparison of the output of the two systems should constitute part of the validation process.

Validation process

1   **Defining the system**
     As the computerised system consists of software, hardware and a process which is to be performed using the software, the first step is to decide what process is to be 'computerised' and how this will broadly be achieved. For example, 'The department wishes to produce patient-specific labels for parenteral nutrition bags using a standardised template.'

2   **Documentation of requirements**
     Once the overall objective of a new system is defined, the exact requirements of what the system will need to achieve in its operating environment is documented in detail via the creation of a 'User Requirements Specification' (URS). This document should take a step-wise approach through the processes which will be performed while using the system in order to identify all possible functionality the end user would like the system to provide. The URS fulfils a number of functions:

     - It gives potential system suppliers a means of understanding what the system must do
     - It forms the basis for all of the validation which follows.

     It can be useful to include a scoring system in the URS to rank functionality by level of importance, as unless a completely bespoke system is being produced it is unlikely that any supplier will be able to meet all of the requirements.

Potential scoring systems include:

- The Acronym 'MoSCoW' – which defines requirements as:
    - Must have (Essential Function)
    - Should have (High Priority but not essential)
    - Could have (Desirable but not necessary)
    - Would like (Would like to see functionality offered in the future)
- A simple assessment of each feature of a system as:
    - Essential
    - Desirable
    - Indifferent.

3   **Assessment of available solutions and suppliers (Design Qualification (DQ))**
The URS should then be sent to potential suppliers to invite them to submit a proposed system which will meet the requirements stated. On receipt of the manufacturer's functional specification or description of the software (where existing software packages are supplied), an assessment should be made to compare how well the features offered by a system meet the requirements laid out in the URS, making use of the scoring systems defined above to aid decision making and allowing a robust choice of supplier.

Once a shortlist of suppliers has been identified, it is essential to assess the competency of the suppliers via supplier assessment or audit depending on:

- The ability of the supplier to demonstrate their quality systems. (Evidence of a robust quality system, e.g. ISO9001 accreditation, may negate the need for full supplier audit.)
- Evidence of strong involvement in an NHS preparation/production environment. (Suppliers with evidence of successful installations in a comparable preparation/ production environment are likely to need less rigorous assessment of competence to meet GMP standards.)

As with all processes, supplier assessment should follow a risk-based approach with levels of scrutiny being dictated by the criticality of the system being offered.

For a bespoke critical system, assessment may take the form of a formal audit of the quality system at a supplier's premises. By contrast, for a computerised system with a proven history of use in a comparable environment, assessment via a questionnaire sent to the supplier (postal audit), or visits to appropriate reference sites may be sufficient.

Implementation of a system from a limited pool of suppliers (or a single vendor)

Where the system is chosen from a limited pool of options (or indeed is the only option available), and has evidence of successful use in a similar NHS pharmacy environment, the URS is still a key document, however it may be possible to draw much of its content from documentation provided by the system vendor, with requirements being based largely on the functionality of the available system.

4   **Installation Qualification (IQ)**
     Once the software is installed, the first step of validation is to ensure that:

- the correct version of the application software is available on all appropriate computers
- the correct version of server software (where applicable) is installed and accessible by the local machines
- users are able to gain access to the software throughout the facility (according to software licence arrangements)
- it is possible to create security accounts for users with access privileges appropriate to their role
- creation of labels, worksheets, reports, and similar system outputs match the standard departmental document format
- creation/alteration of system descriptors match existing hospital ward and department identifiers, as appropriate.

5   **Operational Qualification (OQ)**
     The key functional requirements of the system identified in the URS should undergo a risk assessment process to evaluate which of these functions have the potential to cause a failure of GMP and therefore potential patient harm.

Risk assessment can be performed as follows:

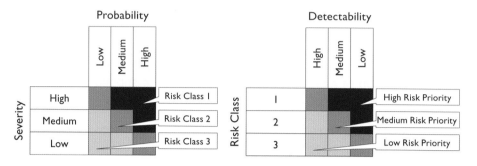

Severity = Impact on Patient Safety, Product Quality and Data Integrity (or other harm)

Probability = Likelihood of the fault occuring

Risk Class = Severity x Probability

Detectability = Likelihood that the fault will be noted before harm occurs

Risk Priority = Risk Class x Detectability

Those areas which have a high risk of failure or a significant impact in the event of failure should be made the subject of a series of test cases written to stress the system in a simulation of 'in-use' conditions in order to prove that the configuration of the system is such that the error/failure either cannot occur or would be readily detected should it ever occur. All test cases should be carried out in triplicate, with a 100% pass rate expected. Any deviation from expected behaviour should be recorded in a deviation report and remedial action taken before the system is put into active use.

6   Performance Qualification (PQ)

PQ is the final step in the initial validation effort and it encompasses testing of the system once it is under actual 'in-use' conditions to ensure that it continues to operate as expected. As a minimum, testing should cover:

- Security – ensure users can only access functions appropriate to their role (ideally an audit trail should be present recording all attempts at access to the system, successful or not)

- System accessibility – ensure that the software remains responsive when in use by several concurrent users

- Data integrity – ensure that information input by one operator can be retrieved by another operator at a later date. Also ensure that changes to data can only be made in appropriate circumstances, and that any such alteration leaves an audit trail which leads back to the user involved.

Choice and content of test cases should be guided by risk assessment of potential failure modes and are likely to be a mixture of tests used during the OQ stage and specific PQ test scripts created to verify functionality of the software in an 'in-use' state (for example, load testing of the system with multiple operators using functions at the same time).

7   **Change control and performance requalification**
Throughout the operational life of the system it is likely that updates to the software will be applied and alterations made to its configuration. Any such changes should be handled through a formal change control mechanism to ensure that changes over time do not cause the system to diverge from its validated state. In response to updates, or to ensure maintenance of the validated state, periodic revalidation is required.

It is suggested that the revalidation interval should be driven by the frequency of updates or changes to the functionality of the system and such revalidation would normally make use of test cases identical to, or based on, the original OQ/PQ documents.

8   **Continuity planning / disaster recovery**
Failure of the hardware or software supporting a computerised system is a very real possibility, resulting in the system becoming unavailable for use. As the function of the computerised system is potentially critical to ensuring GMP compliance, there is a need for a continuity plan to be in place for each computerised system to enable work to continue as promptly as possible following any system failure. Therefore each system should have:

- A method of running the system from backup data which mirrors 'normal' functionality
- An approved written procedure of how to bring the backup system into use
- Documentary evidence that this plan has been tested as effective.

Such capability should, ideally, be written into the URS so that the backup system is an integral part of the overall system and can be tested as such.

9   **System succession planning**
At a point in the future it is likely that current computerised systems will be superseded by newer software, better able to support the processes of the department. It should be borne in mind that any records held solely in electronic form should remain accessible for the expected life of that particular document or data type according to current legal or best practice,

e.g. five years from dispensing for an unlicensed medicine, or five years from the end of the clinical trial for a dispensed medicine governed by Good Clinical Practice (GCP). Where this period exceeds the working life of the system, provision should be made for retaining access to records in a timely fashion. To support this retention, validation activities may be required to ensure:

- Records and data stored in the outgoing system continue to be accessible after retirement of the software

or

- Records and data can be reliably transferred into the new system and continue to be interrogated.

10 Documentation

Once all validation activities are completed, each validated system will have a set of documentation comprising:

- User requirements specification
- Record of risk assessment carried out against requirements
- System Validation Report to include:
    - Detail of IQ test results
    - OQ protocol (comprising a full set of completed test cases)
    - Traceability matrix (tying together risk assessment outcomes with OQ test cases)
    - PQ Protocol (with results of 'in-use' testing performed).
- A system description (essential for critical systems subject to MHRA inspection) detailing:
    - Principles, objectives, and scope of the computerised system
    - System topology (listing PCs, and associated servers, networks etc.)
    - Summary of the auditable critical aspects of the system
    - Security measures (including full listing of current user permissions)
    - Interfaces to other systems

- Record of change control requests relating to the system
- Training records. User training is a key part of any system and records should be kept of all staff trained to use the system and the level of permissions assigned to that user following training.

The validation methods and activities for all computerised systems present in the unit should be detailed in an over-arching 'Computerised System VMP' (CSVMP).

References

European Commission (2015). *The Rules Governing Medicinal Products in the European Union. Volume 4 Good Manufacturing Practice Medicinal Products for Human and Veterinary Use. Annex 11: Computerised Systems.* Available at: *http://ec.europa.eu/health/files/eudralex/vol- 4/annex11_01-2011_en.pdf* (accessed 12 May 2016).

International Society for Pharmaceutical Engineering (ISPE) (2008). *GAMP-5 A Risk-Based Approach to Compliant GxP Computerised Systems.* Available at: *http://www.ispe.org/gamp-good-practice-guides* (accessed 12 May 2016).

Further guidance is available:-
NHS Pharmaceutical Quality Assurance Committee (PQAC) (2015). *Computer systems validation.* 2nd edn.

PART B – 3: TECHNICAL (QUALITY) AGREEMENTS

Introduction

The aim of this support resource is to provide guidance to aseptic units on technical (quality) agreements that are required to define the responsibilities of the unit (the contract giver – CG) and the provider of the service or product that is outsourced (the contract acceptor – CA).

Technical agreements define the responsibilities of both CG and CA with respect to any issue that can impact on product quality, and should be signed off by a person in a "Quality" role. They are different from Service Level Agreements (SLAs), which generally have a financial and legal focus and cover, for example, timeliness of service, period of notice etc. SLAs can be appropriately signed off by procurement personnel.

Technical Agreements (TAs) should be in place, and regularly monitored according to EU GMP (EC 2015), for any outsourced activity or product that can have potential quality implications. For example, TAs should be in place with external providers of the following:

- Cleanroom laundering services
- Cleaning services
- Estates (particularly for Private Finance Initiatives)
- Laboratory services
- Outsourced compounding
- Maintenance services for critical equipment, e.g. auto-compounders, isolators, unidirectional air flow cabinets, computer software, dose calibrators, air handling units
- Temperature monitoring equipment
- Transport.

This list is not exhaustive and serves only to illustrate key services for individual consideration by each aseptic unit. The requirement for a TA is specified in several of the standards in Part A.

The following TA is an example of the style of agreement that is generally considered acceptable. The body of the TA defines clearly its scope, relevant standards, and responsibilities in general terms. The appendix to the TA defines responsibilities in the form of a table, with clarity as to whether the CG or CA is responsible for each aspect. The table should mirror the responsibilities described in general terms in the body of the TA. Other styles of TA may, however, be equally acceptable if they fulfil the same criteria.

References

European Commission (2015). *The Rules Governing Medicinal Products in the European Union. Volume 4 Good Manufacturing Practice Medicinal Products for Human and Veterinary Use. Chapter 7: Outsourced Activities*. Available at: ***http://ec.europa.eu/health/files/eudralex/vol-4/vol4-chap7_2012-06_en.pdf*** (accessed 26 February 2016).

QUALITY TECHNICAL AGREEMENT

FOR THE MANUFACTURE AND DELIVERY OF SUPPLEMENTED PARENTERAL NUTRITION

Between

Name of NHS Organisation (Contract Giver – CG)

And

Name of Supplier (Contract Acceptor – CA)

Validity: This agreement is valid for *[insert suitable timeframe]* after the date of the final signature or earlier if requested by either party

Version:

Reference:

QUALITY TECHNICAL AGREEMENT
For the Manufacture and Delivery of Supplemented Parenteral Nutrition

This Technical Agreement is made between:

Name and Address if NHS Organisation (CG)

and

Name and Address of Supplier (CA)

Production Unit Site Address:

MS number:

This contract is supplemental to any financial agreements and any subsequent agreements, between the two parties and will last for the duration of the agreement. The technical agreement shall be reviewed every *[insert suitable timeframe]* or earlier if requested by either party.

This Technical Agreement is executed in duplicate, all of which shall be deemed to be originals, and all of which shall constitute one and the same Agreement binding upon both parties.

This Quality Technical Agreement shall be effective as of the date of the final signature and shall remain in effect until review or termination.

1. Scope

This agreement defines the roles and responsibilities between CG and CA relating to the manufacture and delivery of unlicensed supplemented parenteral nutrition (PN) for patients under the care of CG.

All parties agree as follows:-

2. Subject of the Agreement

1.   CA is a provider of ready-to-administer supplemented PN which is manufactured according to an agreed specification and delivered to CG.

2.   CA shall manufacture and deliver the products in accordance with this technical agreement and in addition to other financial agreements.

3.   CA is subject to registration and inspection by the competent national authorities and holds the necessary manufacturing licence according to the respective legislation.

CA hereby acknowledges that CG is relying on the skill and experience of CA in the proper manufacture and delivery of the contractual products under this Agreement and CA accordingly warrants to CG that:

■ The product shall be of satisfactory quality and fit for purpose

■ The product shall comply in all respects with order provided by CG.

Both parties will strictly observe the detailed pharmaceutical responsibilities which are specified in Appendix 1 ("Responsibilities").

CG and CA must appoint Contact Persons as named in Appendix 2 ("Contact Persons").

3. Regulatory Information

CA is responsible for ensuring that manufacture and distribution of products meets all current legislation and best practice guidelines.

For the period of the contract, CG will ensure that they hold suitable MHRA approval for the supply of unlicensed supplemented PN.

4. Starting Materials

CA shall source starting materials which possess a UK marketing authorisation or which have been manufactured under a 'manufacturers specials' licence. Materials must be sourced from a bona fide Manufacturer or Wholesaler holding a UK Wholesale Dealer's Authorisation.

5. Manufacture

CA shall provide adequate premises, equipment and staff to satisfactorily carry out the work undertaken. CA shall perform all operations in accordance with Good Manufacturing Practice.

CA shall manufacture the PN in accordance with the specification provided by CG.

CA shall refrain from performing any activities that could adversely affect the quality of the service provided.

6. Quality Control / Assurance

CA must provide sterility assurance of all products purchased by CG. The method to determine sterility assurance must be in line with current Pharmacopoeial requirements and be compliant with current guidance e.g. MHRA Q&As.

CA shall obtain satisfactory stability information for each supplemented PN bag before allocation of an expiry period. This data shall be provided to CG upon request.

Release of each batch of product shall be under the authority of an authorised releasing officer.

CA shall maintain a suitable Pharmaceutical Quality System.

CA acknowledges that CG will perform sample inspection on batches received. Any deficiencies found during sample inspection which relate in some way to the Product supplied by CA will be referred to CA at the earliest opportunity. This may lead to a formal complaint.

CA shall provide Certificates of Conformance for each batch supplied. The Certificate of Conformance shall at a minimum specify:

     a. Name and site of manufacture

     b. Name or description of product

     c. Product Batch or Lot number

     d. Batch size

     e. Storage conditions

     f. Expiry date

     g. Date of manufacture

     h. Statement that the product has been manufactured in compliance to applicable GMP requirements

     i. Name and title of person responsible for the validity of the certificate and the data it contains.

7. Storage and Distribution

CA shall adhere to Good Distribution Practice.

CA shall ensure that product shall be delivered in accordance with agreed procedures and records of delivery and receipt shall be retained by each party to affect a satisfactory audit trail in the event of recall.

CA shall store, handle and distribute the product according to its defined storage conditions.

CA shall be required to provide evidence that the appropriate storage temperatures have been maintained and that all systems have been validated upon request.

CA shall ensure all products are packaged in such a way as to give them adequate protection from damage during transit.

8. Documentation

CA will archive completed documentation according to current regulatory guidance.

9. Change Control

Information related to any planned change to the product, overall process or specification for the product(s) by CA is to be notified to CG in writing at the earliest opportunity and authorised by CG prior to the change being in effect.

It is recognised that problems relating to the supply of starting materials may require urgent action. The substitution of any starting material with an equivalent material that holds a UK marketing authorisation should be notified to CG at the earliest opportunity prior to implementation.

In the event of merger, acquisition or facility closure of CA or any of its agreed subcontractors, CA shall notify CG at least three months before the change is implemented.

CA shall not delegate or sub-contract any of the work entrusted to it under the Contract Agreement without prior evaluation and approval of the arrangements by CG. Any such arrangements made between CA and any approved third party shall ensure that the information relating to this contract is made available and remains confidential in the same way as between CG and CA.

CA shall be responsible for inherent responsibilities of their sub-contractors. Terms of this TA must be adhered to by any approved subcontractor.

10. Unplanned Deviations

Information relating to any major or critical unplanned deviation associated with the individual batch supplied or overall process by CA is to be notified to CG in writing at the earliest opportunity e.g. prior to the product being delivered.

Unplanned deviations which do not directly relate to a contractual product but could impact on the quality of a product purchased by CG should also be reported at the earliest opportunity.

11. Complaints

Any complaint from CG concerning quality of supplied product shall be acknowledged by CA within 24 hours.

A report containing details of the investigation with corrective and preventative actions, as appropriate, shall be forwarded to the CG within ten working days; this may take the form of an interim report if the investigation has not been completed within this timeframe. The CA shall make every effort to complete investigations and provide feedback, including actions assigned, to CG in a timely manner.

Any complaint regarding non-adherence to this TA by either party should be escalated to the line manager of the relevant signatory for this agreement if a satisfactory outcome cannot be achieved by discussion. Ultimately, if a satisfactory outcome still cannot be achieved, financial penalties or termination of the contract may be considered.

12. Recalls and Returns

CA shall notify CG of any recall or near miss (company or MHRA led) relating to contracted products manufactured by CA or starting materials / components which were used in their manufacture.

Recalls and near misses which do not directly relate to a contractual product but could impact on the quality of a product purchased by CG should also be reported at the earliest opportunity.

CA shall co-coordinate and document the recall process. CA is responsible for coordination and disposal of all products returned by CG patients. CA will cooperate with the collection, logging, storage and segregation of any recalled and returned product as required.

13. Audit

CG is responsible for assessing the competence of CA to carry out successfully the work required; this may be through review of a relevant audit performed on behalf of the NHS.

CA shall perform internal audits and perform audits of any outsourced activities.

CG is entitled to audit CA facilities relevant for the manufacture of the contractual products on a bi-annual basis and on specific occasions, e.g. "For-Cause-Audits". Dates for bi-annual audits shall be mutually agreed at least four weeks in advance and For-Cause-Audits one working day in advance.

14. Confidentiality

The information contained in this agreement is confidential and must not be divulged to any other party without the permission of all signatories.

15. Contingency

CA must ensure a robust contingency plan has been arranged to ensure continuity of service in the event that they cannot provide the pre-defined quantities of PN as defined by CG. The use of any sub-contractors must be agreed by CG prior to implementation (see above). Any contingency partner must agree to the terms within this technical agreement.

Final Provision

Amendments of this Quality Technical Agreement and its Appendices may only be carried out by mutual consent and shall be made in writing. Any amendments to the appendices 1-5 may be signed for CG by a responsible Quality representative and, together with the signature of CA, the appendix will be binding upon the parties.

Appendices

Appendix 1	Responsibilities
Appendix 2	List of Sub-contractors
Appendix 3	Technical Agreement Approval
Appendix 4	Key Contact Persons
Appendix 5	Version History

Appendix 1
Responsibilities

	CG	CA	COMMENTS
1. Regulatory Processes			
Hold appropriate 'specials' manufacturing licence of relevant national authority in order to manufacture products as agreed by CG. Comply with any, and all, EU and other local current applicable laws, regulations and guidelines relating to GMP and GDP. CG is to be informed of any changes to licence, outcome of regulatory inspection and any pending regulatory action. Actions to remedy any deficiencies identified by regulatory inspection shall be made available to CG upon request.	✔		
Ensure pharmacovigilance systems are in place to collect and collate information concerning all suspected adverse events / reactions reported to CG.	✔	✔	
Report pharmacovigilance events to CA.	✔		
Ensure competent authorities are notified of all complaints concerning suspected adverse events / reactions / lack of effect according to existing regulations and requirements.	✔	✔	

	CG	CA	COMMENTS
2. Starting / Raw Materials and Excipients			
Purchase sterile materials from bona fide suppliers.	✔		
Assessing the quality of starting materials for use.	✔		
All starting materials are TSE/BSE free.	✔		
Maintain a supplier qualification programme.	✔		
Check that the condition of all containers, closures, seals and labelling of delivered starting materials are satisfactory for use.	✔		
Approval of materials for use.	✔		

	CG	CA	COMMENTS
3. Packaging Material			
Only purchase primary packaging materials from approved suppliers in accordance with a specification.	✔		
Maintain a supplier qualification programme.	✔		
Check that the condition of all packaging material is satisfactory for use.	✔		
Approve packaging for use.	✔		

	CG	CA	COMMENTS

4. Processing

	CG	CA	COMMENTS
Qualification / Validation according to applicable GMP requirements for production equipment, utilities and processes.		✔	
Maintain a suitable environment.		✔	
Maintain a specific batch number system to identify individual products.		✔	
Manufacturing process including all necessary activities.		✔	
In-process checks are performed and are deemed satisfactory.		✔	
Appropriate design and use of manufacturing batch documentation.		✔	
All critical automated processes are fully validated and appropriate for use and meet the requirements of GAMP.		✔	
Ensure that all products are manufactured in accordance with the agreed specification and current legislation.		✔	
Handle medicines with appropriate safety measures.		✔	
Ensure all labelling of products is in compliance with all laws, regulations and guidelines associated with the labelling of unlicensed specials.		✔	

	CG	CA	COMMENTS
5. Stability			
Provide stability data to support the allocated expiry period of the products. Methods to determine product stability shall be in line with current regulatory requirements.		✔	This data shall be made available to CG upon request.

	CG	CA	COMMENTS
6. Sterility			
Provide sterility assurance using methods defined in current guidelines.		✔	
Maintain a suitable system to record, investigate and risk assess all microbiological non-conformances (out-of-limit) results. Implement appropriate corrective and/or preventative actions following the investigation and root cause analysis.		✔	
Assess the potential impact a microbiological non-conformance (isolated result or 'trend') could have on product quality and patient risk, and act accordingly.		✔	
Trend microbiological non-conformances.		✔	
Make available an annual summary of all microbiological non-conformances to CG on request.		✔	

	CG	CA	COMMENTS
6. Sterility (cont.)			
Inform CG of any microbiological non-conformances relating to products received by CG within 48 hours of receipt.		✔	It is recognised that this may be in retrospect. Microbiological non-conformances which do not directly relate to a contractual product but could impact on the quality of a product used by a patient of CG should also be reported. The investigation and any associated corrective and/ or preventative actions shall be made available upon request by CG.

	CG	CA	COMMENTS
7. Product release			
Product release according to agreed criteria.		✔	
Preparation of documentation for release.		✔	
Have satisfactory systems in place that ensures patients only receive released products.		✔	
Released product conforms to order placed by CG.		✔	

	CG	CA	COMMENTS
8. Storage / Distribution			
Qualification / Validation of storage sites for starting materials and products as appropriate.		✔	
Qualification / Validation of transport of the products from place of manufacture to the CG.		✔	
Store all Products and/or starting materials / other ingredients / excipients / auxiliary materials under appropriate conditions in compliance with GMP/GDP requirements and any licence requirements.		✔	
Maintain an audit trail to the patient.	✔	✔	CG to maintain audit trail after receipt of product.
Ensure delivery containers protect the product during delivery and comply with health and safety standards.	✔	✔	
Distribute to the CG in a timely way as described in this technical agreement and other financial agreements.		✔	

	CG	CA	COMMENTS
9. Documentation			
Ensure that prescription forms as well as records of manufacture and distribution are clear, readily available and retained for the period required by current legislation. Records shall ensure the traceability of the origin and destination of Products.		✔	
Ensure that prescription forms are clear and legible.	✔		
Archive documents according to current regulatory guidance.	✔	✔	

PART B – 3: TECHNICAL (QUALITY) AGREEMENTS

	CG	CA	COMMENTS
9. Documentation (cont.)			
Ensure written procedures are available to describe all operations that may affect the quality of the products.	✔		
Maintain complete and accurate records relating to the manufacture, packaging and storage of products supplied.	✔		
Store all documents and records so that they are easily retrievable and stored protected from loss and damage.	✔		
Maintain a record of batch numbers of all starting materials and products manufactured, supplied or returned in the event of a recall.	✔		

	CG	CA	COMMENTS
10. Changes			
Maintain a suitable change control system and communicate all information relating to planned changes with quality implications in writing before implementation.	✔		See above for timelines.
Maintain a suitable unplanned deviation system and communicate all unplanned changes (unplanned deviations excluding microbiological results) deemed to be major or critical. Events shall be reported at the earliest possible opportunity e.g. before delivery of the product.	✔		Unplanned deviations which do not directly relate to a contractual product but could impact on the quality of a product used by a CG patient should also be reported. The investigation and any associated corrective and/or preventative actions shall be made available upon request by CG.

	CG	CA	COMMENTS
10. Changes (cont.)			
Results of any investigation relating to a major or critical unplanned deviation for a contracted product shall be provided in written format to CG within 72 hours of completion.	✔		This investigation must include proposed corrective and/or preventative actions.
No work should be sub-contracted without the prior written agreement of CG.	✔		

	CG	CA	COMMENTS
11. Complaints			
Acknowledge any complaints from CG or patients of CG with quality implications within 24 working hours.	✔		
Investigate and document any complaint relating to the quality of contracted products within 10 days, feedback may be in the form of an interim or final report. This document should include details of all corrective and/or preventative actions as appropriate.	✔		All feedback to be to CG, not to patient.

	CG	CA	COMMENTS
12. Recalls			
In the event of product or any starting materials or components being recalled, arrange for the collection, stocking and segregation of products affected. This also includes products which were manufactured using a recalled starting material or component.	✔		Must comply with timelines as specified in regulations.
Maintain a product recall procedure for use, when it is necessary, to recall a defective product from the market, and test the procedure at least annually.	✔		This also includes products which were manufactured using a recalled starting material or component.

	CG	CA	COMMENTS
12. Recalls (cont.)			
Advise CG if they have received products which are / contain starting materials which are subject to MHRA Drug Alert or Recall.		✔	Must comply with timelines as specified in regulations.
Inform prescribers of any recalls concerning products supplied to patients.	✔		

	CG	CA	COMMENTS
13. Audit			
Provide reasonable access, at agreed pre-determined times, to permit audits of the relevant facilities and documents by CG or the regulatory authorities.		✔	
Undertake the necessary quality audits of CA.	✔		
Undertake the necessary quality audits of subcontractors as required for assurance of this agreement.		✔	
Conduct internal audit in order to monitor the implementation of, and compliance with, GMP and GDP.		✔	
Propose necessary corrective measures following internal audit.		✔	
Make available evidence of adherence to internal audit schedules.		✔	
Make available evidence of closure of external audits and inspections, and the anticipated date of the next MHRA inspection.		✔	
Conduct inspections of, all subcontractors in order to monitor the implementation of, and compliance with, GMP and /or GDP.		✔	

	CG	CA	COMMENTS
14. Training			
Train staff involved in all aspects of the service as appropriate to their role.	✔	✔	This includes training of outsourced contractors.
Ensure staff comply with relevant legislation and NHS requirements concerning both patient and commercial confidentiality e.g. Data Protection Act.	✔	✔	

Appendix 2

List of Subcontractors

e.g. Couriers, Contingency partners and Contract Laboratories

Appendix 3

Technical Agreement Approval

Agreed on behalf of the Contract Giver

Name: _____   Name: _____

Title: _____   Title: _____
           (QA Representative)

Signature: _____   Signature: _____

Date: _____   Date: _____

Agreed on behalf of the Contract Acceptor

Name: _____   Name: _____

Title: _____   Title: _____
           (QA Representative)

Signature: _____   Signature: _____

Date: _____   Date: _____

Appendix 4

Key Contact Persons

Contract Giver

NAME	DESIGNATION	CONTACT NUMBER	E-MAIL

Contract Acceptor

NAME	DESIGNATION	CONTACT NUMBER	E-MAIL

Appendix 5

Version History

VERSION NUMBER	DATE OF AMENDMENT	AMENDMENT(S) MADE

PART B – 4: PRODUCTS FOR SHORT-TERM USE – MAXIMUM SHELF LIFE 24 HOURS

Introduction

As discussed in Part A, Chapter 3, there is an increased risk of microbial contamination of products prepared in uncontrolled environments. There is also an increased risk of medication errors when preparing injections without pharmacy oversight. Hence preparation in pharmacy is preferable.

Previous versions of this text (Beaney 2001, Beaney 2006), referred to conditions that would allow preparation in environments remote from the main pharmacy aseptic unit. This model of preparation is no longer common practice and should be discouraged.

Aseptic products made in pharmacy, including in radiopharmacies, should be prepared in accordance with the standards set down in this handbook. In some circumstances, however, this may not be possible, e.g. delay in re-provision of a unit that no longer complies with the standards, temporarily compromised environmental conditions etc. If risk assessment shows that safety would be increased by continuing to prepare products in pharmacy when the alternative would be preparation in an uncontrolled situation, then the use of a restricted shelf life for products, as described here, may be considered as an interim measure to reduce the risk whilst plans to resume a fully compliant facility are progressed. This should be viewed as a temporary measure – not a permanent solution. In this case, the shelf life of the product should be restricted to 24 hours. The expectation, however, is that the product should be used immediately or, if not, it should be stored at 2-8°C (EMEA 1999), unless detrimental to do so, to reduce possible increased microbial risk.

The following commentary highlights factors for consideration and gives examples of circumstances where a restricted shelf life may be applied to products prepared in pharmacy aseptic units.

Chapter 6 – Formulation, stability and shelf life

The Summary of Product Characteristics (SmPC) recommendations should be followed, where available. For all medicinal products, including radiopharmaceuticals, the shortest possible shelf life consistent with the intended use of the product should be given and, if the standards in Part A have been modified as described here, under no circumstances should a shelf life of 24 hours be exceeded.

Chapter 7 – Facilities and equipment

If the facilities or equipment do not comply with the standards in Part A for any reason, a risk assessment should be undertaken to determine whether continued use (with a restricted shelf life for products) is a safer alternative than preparation in an uncontrolled clinical environment.

Examples of situations where this may be the case are:

- Pharmaceutical isolators failing a leak test
- Laminar flow cabinets with a compromised fan
- Pressure differentials between rooms not being achieved
- Interruption to the air supply out of hours
- Delay in refurbishing an ageing unit.

Chapter 11 – Monitoring

The frequency of monitoring may be more than the minimum requirements set down in Part A, depending upon the circumstances for invoking the reduced shelf life.

Additional considerations for radiopharmaceutical preparation

Radiopharmaceuticals should comply with a number of regulations which occasionally conflict. Regulations that control and limit the handling of radioactive substances result in modifications to procedures, as described here.

The majority of radiopharmaceuticals prepared in unlicensed radiopharmacy units contain the radionuclide ^{99m}Tc technetium, which has a half-life of six hours; thus these (and other short-lived radiopharmacy preparations) can be considered as products for short-term use.

Radiopharmaceuticals that contain a radionuclide with a longer half-life, including Technetium generators, should be handled in accordance with the guidance for aseptic preparation in Part A of this handbook.

Technetium radiopharmaceuticals are prepared using kits and eluates from ^{99m}Tc generators. Whilst the processes are aseptic in nature, and therefore the guidance in this handbook is equally applicable, differences due to the radioactive constraints of starting materials and finished products require additional and/or amended considerations to take this into account.

Three such factors are addressed here:

- Radiation protection
- Shelf life and use of the ^{99}Mo/^{99m}Tc generator
- Shelf life of prepared ^{99m}Tc kits.

Radiation protection

The legitimate use of portable equipment within critical zones, over and above that required for normal aseptic preparation, is necessary for protection of the operator from the gamma (and possibly other) rays emitted from the radionuclide being handled. These items are often transferred into, and retained in, a critical zone for the duration of the working session and may include:

- syringe shields
- vial shields e.g. lead or tungsten pots
- shielded sharps containers
- needle re-sheathing devices (see also Part A, Chapter 10)
- heating blocks
- synthesis units
- radiation monitors
- decontamination equipment.

Risk assessments should be carried out around possible disturbance to unidirectional or turbulent air flow conditions that these additional items may cause in critical zones, and potential microbiological contamination following transfer of these items into critical zones.

It is necessary to undertake transfer validation at regular intervals on all portable equipment, as their exposure to non-sterile conditions due to re-use occurs frequently.

Shelf life and use of the ^{99}Mo/ ^{99m}Tc generator

The generator is a licensed pharmaceutical product and provides a source of sterile sodium pertechnetate solution for the preparation of ^{99m}Tc radiopharmaceuticals from kits using aseptic technique. The generator consists of a sterile column containing the long-lived parent radionuclide molybdenum (^{99}Mo) that is packaged in a multi-component, non-sterile plastic/metal housing and will contain lead or depleted uranium shielding. The column is eluted under aseptic conditions with an eluent (sterile Sodium Chloride Injection 0.9%). Multiple elutions may be made over the shelf life of the generator (up to 3 weeks). The generator is transferred into, and maintained in, an EU GMP Grade A (EC 2015) critical zone for the period of its intended use. The eluent does not contain a preservative.

The following factors need to be considered when using a generator for the preparation of radiopharmaceuticals:

- Following its receipt: transfer of the generator from transport packaging that is likely to be microbiologically contaminated into the EU GMP Grade A (EC 2015) critical zone (this is usually a vertical unidirectional air flow (VUAF) cabinet or negative pressure isolator elution chamber).
  It is recommended that transfer validation of this process is carried out on an annual basis using contact plates and included in a change control if a different supplier is used

- Maintaining EU GMP Grade A (EC 2015) conditions in the critical zone during each elution: this includes when attaching eluent vials, and detaching elution vials, from the column.
  It is recommended that finger/gauntlet dabs and/or settle plates are performed during generator elutions. A settle plate should be located near to the point of elution. A finger/gauntlet dab should be carried out where isolators house the generator. It is also recommended that particle monitoring close to, or at the point of, elution is undertaken during initial commissioning of the isolator or VUAF cabinet, and repeated if the type of generator is changed

- Avoiding inadvertent contamination of the column with disinfectants, particularly with sporicides: this can lead to ^{99m}Tc remaining bound to the column *(UltraTechnekow FM Summary of Product Characteristics 2007).*
  It is recommended that only sterile alcohol wipes are used for surface decontamination of elution vials and that their septa are completely dry before use.

Shelf life of prepared kits

Advice relating to the shelf life, and the subsequent drawing up of radiopharmaceuticals from multi-dose vials in clinical areas outside of pharmacy, is available (UKRG 2012).

References

Beaney AM ed. (2001) on behalf of NHS Quality Control Committee. *Quality Assurance of Aseptic Preparation Services* 3rd edn. London: Pharmaceutical Press.

Beaney AM ed. (2006) on behalf of NHS Pharmaceutical Quality Assurance Committee. *Quality Assurance of Aseptic Preparation Services* 4th edn. London: Pharmaceutical Press.

European Commission (2015). *The rules governing medicinal products in the European Community. Vol IV. Good Manufacturing Practice for medicinal products.* Available at: ***http://ec.europa.eu/health/documents/eudralex/vol-4/ index_en.htm*** (accessed 26 February 2016).

European Medicines Evaluation Agency (EMEA) (1999). *Note for guidance on the maximum shelf life for sterile products for human use after first opening.* CPMP/QWP/159/96. London: Committee for Proprietary Medicinal Products.

UltraTechnekow *Technetium ^{99m}Tc generator Summary of Product Characteristics (SmPC).* Date of partial revision of the text November 2007. Available at: ***http://www.mhra.gov.uk/home/groups/spcpil/documents/spcpil/ con1447998212321.pdf*** (accessed 26 May 2016).

UK Radiopharmacy Group (UKRG) (2012) *Safe drawing up of radiopharmaceuticals in nuclear medicine departments* ***http://www.bnms.org.uk/images/stories/UKRG/UKRG_Drawing_up_Feb-12.pdf*** (accessed 26 May 2016).

PART B – 5: CAPACITY PLANNING – TECHNICAL SERVICES

In order to manage increasing workload within an aseptic unit it is important to have local guidelines on the maximum numbers of items that can safely be prepared, i.e. capacity planning. This involves analysis and decisions to balance capacity in a unit with demand from customers. Units should have sufficient preparation capacity to be able to supply the correct quantity of products at the right time without compromising quality. Capacity planning is used to examine volume and complexity of workload, time available and the staff and facilities required. It is also used to determine contingency strategies to be adopted in the event of inadequate resources, and to determine action to be taken when demands on a unit for products exceeds its safe capacity.

Capacity planning is required to ensure that:

- response/lead times remain within agreed time limits
- quality and safety standards are not compromised
- excessive overtime is not worked or excessive pressure placed on staff
- error and defective product rates do not increase as a result of increased workload.

Capacity planning is a requirement in both licensed and unlicensed units and the Inspectorate of the Medicines and Healthcare products Regulatory Agency (MHRA) have increasingly highlighted this aspect (MHRA 2015). In unlicensed units, particularly those supplying a range of centralised intravenous additive (CIVA) preparations on demand, the workload can be very variable and unpredictable from one day to the next, or even from one hour to the next. In order to manage this type of service a variation of capacity planning termed 'contingency planning' may be used periodically, or continually, to review the situation and take appropriate action based on a risk assessment of the products required and the resources available. Strategic capacity planning is useful when setting up a new service, or developing an existing service, and is based on staff, facilities and workload. Formulae are available to determine the number of staff and facilities required to provide a given workload (Shield 2004). Some of these distinguish between different grades of staff and can hence improve skill mix. They can also allow prediction of the staffing implications of specific increases in workload. However, it should be decided whether these calculations are based on average workload over a given period, or peak workload to meet an infrequent, but predictable, event.

Use of the capacity plan

The MHRA recommend that capacity of an aseptic unit should not exceed 80% (MHRA 2015). This is to allow for variation in demand on the service and also for any associated essential tasks such as quality assurance (QA) / quality management (QM) activities and training. It is unlikely that management would be happy for units to be constantly underused by 20%. An alternative approach is to remove time for essential tasks from the available staff time before preparing the capacity plan. Aseptic units could then aim for 100% capacity while still allowing time for associated tasks to be completed. Limits could be set to allow for the fluctuation in demand, with units aiming to work at 90 – 110% of capacity. Any breach of these limits for more than a specific time period should trigger actions previously agreed with senior pharmacy management, as work above 100% means that time is being taken from the protected periods built into the plan. These protected periods are essential for specialist duties. An escalation mechanism to senior hospital managers should be agreed so that if limits are exceeded for more than a specified time, e.g. three months without an identified self-limiting reason then plans should be in place for managing the situation, e.g. by reducing workload, implementing contingency plans, or increasing staff.

The capacity plan, once developed, should become a live document which is reviewed when there are significant changes to supply and demand, or at least annually. Compliance with the plan should be assessed monthly, preferably within a management review meeting, and any increase in workload exceeding 100% of the calculated maximum should be discussed. Any increase in workload to the point at which quality and safety standards would be compromised should urgently be discussed with senior pharmacy and hospital management. Any proposed changes should be evaluated through the change control system. The defined capacity should only be exceeded infrequently, and senior pharmacy management approval sought through the use of the planned deviation system.

The capacity plan should be part of, or referenced in, the overall organisation's aseptic preparation policy and should be agreed and signed by the Chief Pharmacist and hospital management.

Unplanned breaches in maximum capacity should be raised as a deviation and discussed at senior pharmacy management level, with strategies put in place to mitigate the risk of these breaches in the future.

If the capacity plan defined workload volumes are regularly exceeded, this should be documented on the hospital's risk register and measures put in place to address the issues urgently.

Factors in capacity planning

1   **Workload**
    The staff time required to prepare different types of product, using different processing methods, varies significantly; for example, making additions to a premixed parenteral nutrition (PN) bag compared with compounding a similar bag from all the basic ingredients or preparing a chemotherapy regimen for a clinical trial compared with a similar non-trial product.
    The effect of preparing multiple items should also be taken into account. There could be a significant difference in the time taken to prepare a number of items at the same time when compared with preparing the same number of the same items individually.

    For aseptic preparation units with a complex mix and high volume of products, assessing workload changes (and calculating the staffing resources required) is simplified if standard work units (reflecting 'activity' time) are assigned to each product category or task. These units should be applied not only to those direct activities needed to make a product but also indirect activities such as ordering, record keeping, equipment monitoring and maintenance, cleaning, environmental monitoring, etc.

2   **Staffing**
    In order to assess the staffing resources required and available, their number, grade and status should be identified:

    - numbers – employed, available for work in aseptic unit
    - grade – pharmacists, technicians, assistants
    - status – permanent, rotational, trainee
    - capability – depending on amount of training and experience of working in the unit.

3   **Facilities**
    Capacity of equipment in terms of time available for isolators, unidirectional air flow cabinets, checking benches, etc., should be determined and any rate-limiting steps identified. Space availability should also be taken into account, e.g. storage capacity in refrigerators and freezers.

4   Quality Management (QM)

The time taken to carry out QM activities should be included in the capacity plan. Resources required for QM activities should not be seen as less important than those required for product preparation.

Examples of QM activities include:

- Generating and reviewing standard operating procedures
- Generating new master worksheets and labels
- Deviations, change control, CAPA (corrective and/or preventative action), investigation of product failures
- Reviewing environmental monitoring data
- Quality meetings
- Equipment, operator and process validation
- Internal and external audits
- Capacity planning
- Trend monitoring
- External meetings
- Quality monitoring of maintenance and contractors.

Devising a formula

1   Time

The time taken for the preparation of any product can be split into three steps:

(i)   Fixed time per session. This could include preparation of the workspace, daily monitoring, gowning in clean room clothing, etc.

(ii)   Fixed time per item or set of items. This could include preparation of the labels and worksheet, collection of ingredients, transfer sanitisation of ingredients, time to dry after wiping, (especially with aqueous sporicides – see Part A, Chapter 12) hatch lockout time, in-process checks, final check, product approval.

(iii) Manipulation time per item. This is the actual time taken to prepare a specific product. To simplify counting, locally determined standard time values can be assigned to each product type, e.g.:

parenteral nutrition bag - 20 minutes*
simple cytotoxic item - 10 minutes*
complex cytotoxic item - 20 minutes*.

2 Staff

The grade of staff used to carry out each step can be identified and locally determined time values linked to staff grade, e.g.:

Fixed time* per session
- 1 hour of assistant time
- 30 minutes technician time.

Fixed time per item or set of items
- 30 minutes of assistant time
- 10 minutes technician time
- 15 minutes pharmacist time.

Manipulation time per item
- standard time value of technician time.

A set of items may be manipulated simultaneously and this should be taken into account.

*Standard time values and staffing times are for illustrative purposes only. They are not fixed and should be determined locally for each unit.

3 Equipment

If equipment rather than staff is the limiting factor, then time per item (e.g. cytotoxic item in isolator) can be calculated and used instead of staff time.

4 Quality Management

QM tasks should be included within any calculations and appropriate resources assigned to complete the required activities.

The time taken to perform each activity should be assigned per staff grade and multiplied by the number of times that activity is performed each year to give the total resources required for that activity. Totalling these required resources will give the total time required to effectively maintain the quality system.

Care should be taken to ensure QM activities are not also included in resource allocation for preparation to avoid double counting.

Calculation of total time

The total time required to prepare a set number of items can be calculated by relating the three preparation steps to staff grade and number of items produced, for example:

(i) Fixed time per session multiplied by number of sessions per month would estimate total sessional time required for technicians and assistants.

(ii)   Fixed time per product multiplied by the approximate number of products prepared per month could estimate total product time required for assistants, technicians and pharmacists.

(iii)   Standard time values per item multiplied by the approximate number of various items could estimate the total manipulation time required for technicians. By adding the total time in the previous three steps, the time required for the three staff groups per month can be calculated.

Time available
The total time worked by staff members of each grade in one month can be calculated. Time for annual leave (A/L), bank holidays, percentage capability per staff member in training, indirect activities (e.g. ordering, planned preventative maintenance, environmental monitoring), etc., can be estimated and subtracted from the total monthly time. The time and grade of staff required to undertake QM activities should be calculated, as described earlier. This time should also be subtracted from the total monthly time to give the time available. It is important that time is allowed to adequately provide the professional aspects of the service, not merely a technical supply service. Additional factors to be taken into account include specific items for radiopharmacy, for example.

Calculating capacity – an example

To determine the capacity used in an aseptic unit, the time required for the preparation of each type of item should be calculated and a spreadsheet created. The workload for a specific month should then be counted and added to the spreadsheet to give the total time needed for aseptic preparation in a specific month for all staff grades (see Table B5.1).

Table B5.1
Aseptic unit workload recording

	ACCOUNTABLE PHARMACIST	PHARMACIST	SENIOR TECHNICIAN	TECHNICIAN	ASSISTANT
Chemotherapy					
Monthly items .....**1,000**..... × 7P + 17T + 8A					
(Time for pharmacist checking, technician setting up, assistant transfer decontamination.)		7,000		17,000	8,000
No of Sessions .....**40**..... × 30T (Time to clean isolator, change gloves, environmental monitoring of isolator.)				1,200	
Cytotoxic work units .....**3,680**..... × 3T					
(Cytotoxic work units are units of time to prepare chemotherapy, with 1 item being the quickest item e.g. methotrexate syringe.) *				11,040	
Parenteral nutrition and CIVA					
No of sessions .....**20**..... × 30T (Time to clean isolator, change gloves, environmental monitoring of isolator.)				600	

	ACCOUNTABLE PHARMACIST	PHARMACIST	SENIOR TECHNICIAN	TECHNICIAN	ASSISTANT
Parenteral nutrition bag (adult) .....**100**..... x 10P + 45T + 15A		1,000		4,500	1,500
Parenteral nutrition bag (neonate) .....**30**..... x 10P + 40T + 10A		300		1,200	300
CIVA (simple).....**125**..... x 3P + 20T + 6A		375		2,500	750
CIVA (complex) .....**40**..... x 5P + 23T + 8A		200		920	320
Totals		8,875		38,960	10,870

P = Number of minutes of pharmacist time T= Number of minutes of technician time A= Number of minutes of assistant time

* By allocating work units to a chemotherapy item, the complexity of the item is taken into consideration. An increase in complex items will then have a greater impact on capacity than an increase in simple items. Parenteral nutrition and CIVA items have manipulation time in isolator included in the formula. This is because there is often less variation in time to prepare a PN bag or CIVA item. **Note these timings are examples only. Units should use locally determined timings.**

The time available should be calculated. This time should be calculated in minutes per month (after removing average annual leave and bank holidays). If a staff member is in training then a percentage capability should be applied. This should be determined locally but see Table B5.2 for suggested guidance values. If a staff member has specific duties other than aseptic preparation, such as QA/QM/environmental monitoring/ cleaning, then this time should be removed. (see Table B5.3). The time available divided by the time used for each staff grade will give the capacity used for that particular month. (see Table B5.4).

Table B5.2
Guidance on percentage capability for assistants / technicians (Bands 3-5) in training

MONTHS INTO TRAINING	STAFF WHO HAVE NEVER WORKED IN ANY ASEPTIC SUITE PERCENTAGE CAPABILITY	STAFF WHO HAVE PREVIOUSLY HAD ASEPTIC EXPERIENCE ELSEWHERE PERCENTAGE CAPABILITY
1	0	0
2	20	30
3	30	50
4	50	70
5	70	85
6	80	100
7	90	
8	100	

Table B5.3
Time available per staff group

	TIME AVAILABLE
Accountable Pharmacist	8,212 minutes 50% QA/QM/Clinical/Managerial = 4,106 minutes available
Pharmacist	Part time 3 days per week 60% of 8,212 = 4,927 minutes 10% of role is training = 4,434 minutes available
Senior Technician	8,212 minutes 40% of role is managerial & IT = 4,927 minutes available

	TIME AVAILABLE
Technician (Band 3-5)	2 x 8,212 minutes but lose 0.45wte in chemotherapy liaison & QC roles 1.55 x 8,212 = 12,729 mins 3 x 8,422 minutes but lose 0.4wte as 2 partly trained 2.6 x 8,422 = 21,897 Total technicians = 34,626 minutes available
Assistant (Band 2)	2 x 8,422 but lose 0.6wte in QC / cleaning 1.4 x 8,422 = 11,791 minutes available

wte – whole time equivalent

To calculate number of minutes per staff member per month

$$\frac{((37.5 \text{ hours} \times 52 \text{ weeks}) - (\text{number of days A/L} + \text{B/H in hours})) \times 60}{12}$$

27 days A/L = 8,422 mins/month
29 days A/L = 8,363 mins/month
33 days A/L = 8,212 mins/month

Table B5.4
Percentage capacity used

	TIME AVAILABLE	TIME USED	PERCENTAGE CAPACITY USED
Accountable Pharmacist	4,106 minutes		See combined figures in box below
Pharmacist	4,434 minutes Combined pharmacists 8,540 minutes	8,875 minutes	104%
Senior Technician	4,927 minutes		See combined figures in box below
Technician (Band 3-5)	34,626 minutes Combined technicians 39,553 minutes	38,960 minutes	99%
Assistant (Band 2)	11,791 minutes	10,870 minutes	92%

The capacity used per month can be trended graphically in order that any sustained increase or decrease in workload can be seen (see example in Figure B5.1).

Figure B5.1
Percentage capacity used

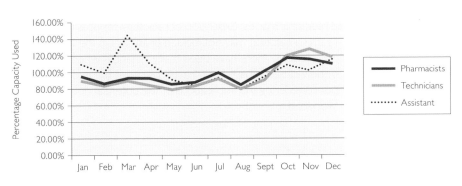

Calculation of extra staff required for an increase in workload

In order to calculate extra staff required for a planned increase in workload, or to bid for staff retrospectively, the required time of the workload increase should be determined. The total time worked by 1 whole time equivalent (WTE) of each grade in one month, minus an allowance for annual leave and bank holidays should be calculated. The number of extra products should then be fed through the total time calculation described above (removing parts of the calculation such as fixed time per session if no extra sessions are required). The total calculated time required per staff grade should then be divided by the time available per 1 WTE to give the number of whole time equivalents of each grade of staff required to prepare a set number of items. Using a formula such as this, the effect of any change in staffing or increase in workload on capacity can easily be determined. In order to assess whether sufficient resources have been available to meet workload over a period of time, quantitative indicators can be used including overtime worked, response times, error rates and product defects. These indicators should be monitored over time to ensure capacity plans remain valid.

Capacity planning for radiopharmacy

This has been described elsewhere (UKRG 2009) but has many similarities with the processes described above. Additional guidance is provided for the professional duties, radiation protection, transport and procurement activities that most radiopharmacy managers and senior radiopharmacy staff routinely undertake.

As radiopharmacies have preparation sessions concentrated at the beginning of the day, staffing pressures can be more difficult to manage than for other types of aseptic activity. Also, capacity issues are more likely to be related to maintaining the pharmaceutical quality system.

Additionally, it should be noted that due to the management structures that exist for many pharmacy-led radiopharmacies, expansion of radiology services (for example, an additional gamma camera) may not include pharmacy in the important initial business planning. Historically there have been many instances where purchasing contracts for new cameras have been hastily placed at the end of the financial year without considering the implications of the potential doubling of the radiopharmacy workload.

Contingency planning

Contingency planning can be used when the workload is likely to exceed the planned capacity of a unit. It can also be used for unforeseen emergencies or sudden events. This may be as a result of sudden, unpredictable peaks in activity, equipment failure or staff shortage. It is hoped that this would not be used regularly. Any use of contingency should be documented through both change control and the deviation reporting systems. The Chief Pharmacist should be aware of any use of contingency (see Part A, Chapter 5). Different strategies may be used depending on the type of contingency:

Sudden events (Self-limiting to a few hours or days)

1   Prioritise the work based on the risk assessment of each product or type of product. Concentrate available resources on those products which have the highest risk weighting in relation to NPSA Patient Safety Alert 20 (NPSA 2007).

2   Consider the urgency of each product. Identify any which can be deferred to later in the day or the next day.

3   Discuss with clinicians whether a ready-prepared alternative can be used if available. (Liaise with procurement colleagues.)

4   Defer some activities not directly connected to product preparation to another day.

5   Transfer suitably competent staff from another section of the aseptic unit temporarily to deal with the peak.

6   Ask staff to extend their working hours temporarily.

7   If the preparation of the product has to take place in a clinical area, ensure that the correct equipment and information is available for it to be prepared as safely as possible. (NPSA 2007, *NHS Injectable Medicines Guide*.)

Foreseen events (Over several days or weeks, e.g. long term sickness, equipment awaiting repair, etc.). As above plus the following:

1   Try to anticipate; prepare some doses in advance up to a 7-day limit, dependent on stability.

2   Liaise with neighbouring hospitals to see if they are able to provide any of the required products.

3   Liaise with neighbouring hospitals to see if it would be possible to use any spare facilities.

4   Purchase some products from a manufacturing unit with a 'Specials' Manufacturing Licence in consultation with procurement colleagues.

5   Investigate temporary loan of a piece of equipment.

6   Temporarily increase staff by secondment from another area of the pharmacy, assess competence and train if necessary. (However, the impact of additional staff on environmental controls, e.g. particle counts should be borne in mind.)

Outsourcing

Outsourcing can be a useful way to deal with workload pressures, with many companies with 'Specials' manufacturing licences offering dose-banded ready-to-use chemotherapy syringes, or bespoke PN bags. Although purchasing these products will reduce the preparation workload in the aseptic unit, the workload associated with dispensing the products is likely to remain and should be included in the capacity plan. Additionally, the work relating to the writing and monitoring of Technical Agreements (see also Part B – 3) with a supplier, and the ongoing monitoring and quality control of the received product, is not inconsiderable and should be included in any workload and capacity calculations. Care should be taken to ensure that time for these activities is linked to the appropriate staff group.

Specimen format of a capacity plan for aseptic preparation unit in hospital X

Current facilities, staffing and activity

Example:

Current facilities: 1-2 glove negative pressure isolator

1-2 glove positive pressure isolator

Current staffing: 1.0 WTE Accountable Pharmacist (permanent)

1.0 WTE Band 6 technician (permanent) for service management

0.5 WTE Band 4 technician (rotational) for total PN

0.7 WTE Band 5 technician (rotational) for cytotoxic reconstitution

0.5 WTE Band 2 assistant for sanitisation of items.

0.1 WTE domestic services (cleaning)

[Insert a plan of aseptic facilities here]

Current activity:	4,000 chemotherapy items per annum
	700 PN bags per annum.
Peak activity negative isolator:	Tuesday afternoon – lung cancer clinics
	Wednesday/Thursday – general oncology clinic
Peak activity positive isolator:	Friday afternoon – PN preparation for weekend

Current capacity status: Under capacity most days with respect to isolator time, but owing to unpredictable nature of requests, capacity is often reached at peak activity times.

Hours of service: Monday-Friday 0900-1700 hours

Type of products available: PN and chemotherapy

Prescriptions for PN: Must be received before 1400 hours

Prescriptions for chemotherapy: Pharmacy must be notified before 1530 hours.

Standards for service provision to the wards

Parenteral nutrition
Wards will receive compounded PN bags from pharmacy for patients who have had PN prescribed for that night via the '5 p.m. porter'. PN for Saturday and Sunday will be sent to the ward on those days before 1700 hours.

Chemotherapy
All outpatient prescriptions receive priority as patients are scheduled every 30 minutes. Wards will be given notice of when chemotherapy for in-patients will be prepared. Pharmacy will contact the ward when the prescription is ready for uplift. Pharmacy will endeavour to meet the needs of all wards and patients but thought must be given to appropriate scheduling of patients.

Activity limits

Maximum no. of PN patients/day: 6

Maximum no. of chemotherapy patients/day: 20 simple or 10 complex regimens.

[List regimes/preparations and category here as an appendix]

1   The activity limits stated are based on timed activities performed by trained and validated staff.

2   Allowances for breaks, annual leave, training, cleaning, environmental monitoring and routine maintenance are built in to these activity limits.

3   These limits are based on all facilities being operational and all trained staff present.

Contingency plans if facilities fail

Identify suitable backup units in advance when preparing the capacity plan. Establish suitable Service Level and Technical Agreements with them to ensure that sufficient alternative capacity exists and is able to respond in case of urgent need.

Adult parenteral nutrition

1   Use product-licensed standard bags.

2   Order from compounding unit with ML 'Specials'.

Chemotherapy

1   Purchase from manufacturing unit with ML 'Specials' where possible.

2   Introduce dose banding together with the purchase of standard dose syringes, with appropriate quality input.

3   Liaise with neighbouring hospital to make use of facilities to prepare items not available from other manufacturers.

Contingency plans for sudden peak in activity

Adult parenteral nutrition

1   Identify stable patients and shift preparation to morning session if possible.

2   Transfer suitable patients to standard product-licensed bags.

3   Prioritise patients who need the service most.

4   Order from ML 'Specials' unit if patient has long-term requirements.

Chemotherapy

1   Defer doses for in-patients to the next day – prioritise outpatients.

2   Defer weekly or monthly environmental monitoring activities to another day.

3   If peak anticipated – try to prepare some doses in advance.

4   If long-term – look to dose band and purchase syringes for certain regimes from a licensed facility with appropriate quality input, e.g. specification.

5   Use overtime for short-term until solution found. (Ensure that suitable arrangements are included in contracts of employment.)

Contingency plans for staff shortage

Facility will be able to accommodate some activity, but this will be less than the stated activity limit.

1   Plan as for sudden peak activity.

2   All staff called on to work in an aseptic unit should be trained to an acceptable level to undertake any given task.

3   If staff can be obtained to work in aseptic preparation unit, efficiency may still be compromised if the staff brought in are relatively inexperienced and require a high level of supervision.

4   If the Accountable Pharmacist is absent a suitable, trained, designated deputy should supervise activities for that day or session. If there are no suitable Authorised Pharmacists available, the Chief Pharmacist should be contacted to decide on an appropriate course of action.

New services and clinics requiring pharmacy support

A clinician wishing to establish a service within the hospital which may regularly, or occasionally, draw on pharmacy aseptic services, should speak to the Accountable Pharmacist and Chief Pharmacist to ensure that the service can be accommodated. Any additional activity requested by clinicians should be supported by funding of the additional capacity required to provide the service. This applies to both new requests for services, and extension to existing levels of service. Capacity may be expanded by recruitment of additional staff, purchase of new equipment, or extension to the hours or days services are provided. When additional services are agreed it is important to understand the anticipated demand, and to monitor the level of activity, to ensure the resources provided for that part of the service are not regularly exceeded.

Other information to be included in capacity plan

1   Detail methodology of determining real preparation times and assigning standard work units.

2   List products or regimes with assigned standard work units.

3   Strategies and actions to be taken if the demands on the aseptic preparation facilities exceed the maximum safe activity level. This should include when to escalate to the Chief Pharmacist and the mechanism for him/her to escalate further to Board level within the organisation. The use of change control and planned deviation should also be included.

4   The frequency of review of the capacity plan (at least annually).

5   The frequency of monitoring of the capacity plan (e.g. monthly during management review meetings).

6   Management approval, both within pharmacy and by hospital management.

References

UK Radiopharmacy Group (UKRG) (2009). *A Capacity Planning Toolkit for Radiopharmacy Services in the UK.* Available at: ***http://www.bnms.org.uk/images/stories/downloads/documents/ukrg_capacity_planning_2009.pdf*** (accessed 18 July 2016).

Medicines and Healthcare products Regulatory Agency (MHRA) (2015). *Questions and Answers for Specials Manufacturers.* London: MHRA. Available at: ***https://www.gov.uk/government/publications/guidance-for-specials-manufacturers*** (accessed 19 February 2016).

National Patient Safety Agency (NPSA) (2007). *Patient Safety Alert. Promoting Safer use of Injectable Medicines.* NPSA 2007/20. London: National Patient Safety Agency.

NHS Injectable Medicines Guide (Medusa) [online]. Available at: ***http://medusa.wales.nhs.uk*** (accessed 19 May 2016).

Shield K (2004). Capacity Planning for Chemotherapy. *Pharm J* 272: 61-62.

PART B – 6: ADVANCED THERAPY MEDICINAL PRODUCTS (ATMPs)

Introduction

Advanced Therapy Medicinal Products (ATMPs) are new and innovative medicinal products based on genes (gene therapy), cells (cellular therapy) and tissues (tissue engineering). Advanced therapies such as these offer the potential for groundbreaking treatments for a wide variety of indications. As such, they have massive potential for both patient benefit and for the pharmaceutical industry. It is essential, as treatments develop and progress, that the pharmacy profession is aware of the requirements for the handling and preparation of ATMPs, and that appropriate facilities are planned for the future.

Cell-based medicinal products cover a wide range of cell therapies, including somatic cell and tissue engineered products that have been manufactured from a patient's own cells (autologous), donor cells (allogenic) or animal cells (xenogenic). Cells, in these circumstances, are classed as medicinal products because they have undergone substantial manipulation or because they are being used to perform a different essential function from that where they originated (non-homologous use).

Tissue engineered products are developed with the aims of repairing, regenerating or replacing various tissue defects.

Gene therapy medicinal products contain genes, administration of which into the human body produce a therapeutic, prophylactic or diagnostic effect via the expression of inserted recombinant nucleic acid.

Gene therapy can be divided into two main categories – gene addition to augment a defective gene, or to deliver a gene with a new function. For gene therapy to be successful, a therapeutic gene must be delivered to the nucleus of a target cell where it can be expressed as a therapeutic protein.

Genes are delivered to target cells by vectors in a process called gene transfer. Gene transfer vectors can be broadly divided into non-viral and viral systems. Nonviral vectors, such as liposomes, have so far shown limited efficacy. Genetically modified (GM) viruses have proved to be the most efficient way of delivering genes. Viruses are merely genetic information protected by a protein coat. They have a unique ability to enter (infect) a cell, deliver viral genes to the cell, and use the host cell machinery to express those genes. A variety of viruses have been used as vectors, including retroviruses, herpes simplex viruses and adenoviruses.

Most viral vectors used are "replication–defective"; they have been genetically modified to ensure removal of the viral genes required to form new viral particles, or revert back to a pathogenic virus. The deleted genes are replaced with a therapeutic gene, thus allowing the delivery and expression of the therapeutic gene without subsequent spread of the virus to surrounding cells. Future gene therapy vectors will be able to replicate under certain conditions. There are potential infectious hazards with gene therapy which include possible transmission of the vector to hospital personnel.

ATMPs may in the future incorporate as an integral part of the product, one or more medical devices in which case they are referred to as "combined advanced therapy medicinal products".

Regulation of ATMPs

Within the European Union, ATMPs are regulated via *Regulation (EC) No 1394/2007 ("The ATMP Regulation")*. This requires that all substances that meet the definition of a medicinal product, as defined in *Directive 2001/83/EC,* and are classified as ATMPs are regulated through the centralised European marketing authorisation (MA) route. The ATMP Regulation includes guidance on what is classified as an ATMP, and specific confirmation should also be sought on a case-by-case basis from the European Medicines Agency (EMA). In reality, at this time, there are a very few ATMPs with Marketing Authorisations and it is therefore most likely that pharmacists will come across advanced therapy investigational medicinal products (ATIMPs) as part of a clinical trial. In this situation, pharmacists should be aware that aseptic pharmacy facilities may not be suitable to be used to prepare ATIMPs for administration as this often requires specialist staff and dedicated cell therapy facilities. Any processing categorised as substantial manipulation by the MHRA, or where the ATIMP is for non-homologous use, will be classified as manufacture and will need to be performed in a specialist manufacturing unit holding a Manufacturer's and Import Authorisation – Investigational Medicinal Products (MIA(IMP)).

Due to the nature of the products and starting materials handled, hospitals should recognise that in many cases it will not be possible to handle these products in existing aseptic facilities and investment in dedicated, purpose designed facilities will be needed.

Advances in regenerative medicine, genetic engineering and recombinant deoxyribonucleic acid (DNA) technology have led to an increase in the number of biotechnology products reaching clinical trials. Manipulations which involve more than solely reconstituting clinical trial products in order to administer them are covered by *The Medicines for Human Use (Clinical Trials) Regulations 2004.* This process will require the manufacturing site to hold an MIA (IMP) from MHRA and QP certification (release) will be required. A suitably detailed Technical Agreement with the sponsor will need to be in place and the manufacturer will need to have access to all the information required for the product specification file, including a copy of the Clinical Trial Authorisation (CTA).

Legal basis for ATMPs

In the UK there are currently two mechanisms by which ATMPs can be made as unlicensed medicinal products. The first is the MHRA's Manufacturers Specials licence which is widely used by NHS Pharmaceutical Manufacturing Units for traditional pharmaceuticals; the second mechanism is an exemption to the need for a MA as provided for in Article 28 of the ATMP Regulation known as the "hospital exemption". Currently the most common regulatory route in the UK is to manufacture under a Specials licence.

The hospital exemption applies to "any ATMP as defined in *Regulation (EC) No 1394/2007,* which is prepared on a non-routine basis according to specific quality standards, and used within the same member state in a hospital under the exclusive professional responsibility of a medical practitioner, in order to comply with an individual medical prescription for a custom-made product for an individual patient."

In the UK, both of these mechanisms for the production of unlicensed ATMPs are regulated by the MHRA and require the appropriate licence.

Due to the very specialist nature of many of these products it is very unlikely that a pharmacy facility will be taking full control of all aspects of the preparation process, and many other specialist professionals will be involved at various stages. However, it is important that an appropriate level of pharmaceutical input is maintained, especially with regards to pharmaceutical Quality Assurance resources, to ensure that facilities and processes operate in compliance with EU Good Manufacturing Practice (GMP) (EC 2015) and with an effective Pharmaceutical Quality System in place (see Part A, Chapter 8). This should also include the provision of appropriate levels of GMP training for other professionals involved in the preparation process. For licensed facilities handling ATMP agents, compliance with EU GMP Annex 2 (EC 2015) will be required.

Technical and Service Level agreements will need to be in place to achieve this to ensure that pharmacy has the appropriate oversight of how these medicinal products are being supplied (see Part B – 3), and so that pharmacy can fulfil its Good Clinical Practice (GCP) responsibilities where the ATMPs is being used in a clinical trial.

Due to the complex nature of these products and processes, a number of other regulatory bodies may also be involved.

Human Tissues are regulated by the Human Tissue Authority (HTA) under *The Human Tissue (Quality and Safety for Human Application) Regulations 2007.* If human embryos are used, the Human Fertilisation and Embryology Authority (HFEA) will also be involved.

If a product containing human tissue is not considered as an ATMP by the MHRA, it will be entirely regulated by the HTA. If it is classified as an ATMP, the HTA regulatory role will only cover the donation, procurement and testing of human cells.

Hence, if an autologous cellular product is to be manufactured, the regulation of the process of collection of the raw material (often the patient's blood) is undertaken by the HTA. However, when this blood is subsequently used as a starting material, the MHRA regulates the production and release of the final product as it is then classed as a medicine.

Pharmacists should seek to engage with the HTA Designated Individual for their organisation to ensure that all advanced therapy IMPs are identified and subject to appropriate pharmaceutical governance.

ATMPs could consist of, or involve the use of, genetically modified organisms (GMOs). Handling of these organisms could also fall under the requirements of *The Genetically Modified Organisms (Contained Use) Regulations 2014* (regulated by the Health and Safety Executive) and/or the *Directive 2001/18/EC (Deliberate Release)*(regulated by the Department of Environment, Food and Rural Affairs).

Advice should be sought from the Health and Safety Executive (HSE) to determine under which Directive the product falls, and any appropriate authorisations required.

In reality, it can be seen from the above that it is not possible for an unlicensed NHS aseptic unit to be involved in manufacturing any ATMP products. All products under the ATMP classification require manufacture under an MS, MIA(IMP) or the hospital exemption of the ATMP Regulation, all of which are regulated by the MHRA. However, if a reconstitution or thawing step is required prior to administration, risk assessment will provide the most appropriate environment for this and this could be in an unlicensed unit, depending on the product and facilities available. This would need to be assessed on a case-by-case basis. At this time, short shelf lives often dictate the need for this activity to occur in the clinical area.

For gene therapies, although *The Genetically Modified Organisms (Contained Use) Regulations 2014* do not refer to GMP standards (EC 2015), it is important to stress that any preparation of medicinal products containing gene therapy agents must comply with GMP requirements. Therefore any guidance on the handling of gene therapy agents must always be undertaken in conjunction with regards to the standard provisions of GMP.

GMOs may be classified as class 1 (low risk) to class 4 (high risk) human pathogen or biological agents. Containment level 1 is required for class 1 agents and containment level 4 for class 4 agents.

All current trials involve Class 1 or 2 agents and, in both of these cases, GMP requirements are much more stringent with respect to facilities, containment and systems of work. The principle should be applied that, where the requirements of GMP are more demanding than those for containment, the GMP requirements must always take precedence. Where an assessment of GMP and containment needs for a specific product show contradictory requirements, a formal documented risk assessment should be undertaken to determine the path of minimal risk to product, patient, operator and environment.

Where a risk assessment has shown that it is feasible to prepare an ATMP, implementation should be facilitated using change control. Where a risk assessment is conducted, appropriate clinical trials colleagues should be involved as risks will cover the complete pathway of the product within the hospital i.e. from receipt to administration.

An impact assessment should be documented and will need to consider the following categories.

a) Facilities
Ideally, gene therapy products should not be manipulated in clinical areas because of the uncertain effects of specific genes on normal human cells, the potential for operator sensitisation on repeated exposure, and the potentially infective nature of some products. Consideration has to be given to protect both the product and the staff handling these agents. A risk assessment should be made for each product, with input from the lead investigator or the organisation's biological safety officer, as they should have a good understanding of molecular biology and virology.

Plasmid DNA and DNA complexes may be manipulated in existing non-cytotoxic aseptic facilities, provided that adequate segregation from other products is achieved by process control and the application of validated cleaning procedures. The main hazard associated with these products is the theoretical risk of immune sensitisation due to their proteinaceous nature. To date this has not been a problem in clinical practice, however.

Viral vectors can be either replication deficient or replicating, and should therefore be considered as infective and be manipulated accordingly. Most gene therapy agents in clinical trials require containment level 1 or 2 facilities. Containment level 2 facilities should be planned in units for the future that would enable the handling of class 2 replicating vectors. Unless specific safety information data indicates a low level of hazard, the following minimum handling requirements should be applied:

- A dedicated negative pressure isolator or Class II microbiological safety cabinet should be used to protect the handler
- The room should be positive in pressure to protect the product, and should be dedicated to the handling of gene therapy agents. This would enable containment level 2 vectors to be handled.

Higher containment levels may require reconsideration of the classic pressure gradients seen in pharmacy aseptic units. A typical design of this sort may see the isolator / safety cabinet in a HEPA filtered room at a lower than ambient pressure, surrounded by classified rooms at a higher than ambient pressure. Airflow pattern and visualisation is of high importance when considering such a design.

Any departures, such as this, from conventional cleanroom design should be subject to the decision of a formal documented risk assessment at the stage of producing the User Requirements Specification.

Consideration may also be given to the use of non-recirculating air handling systems dedicated to that facility only at higher levels of containment

If future trials involve organisms above level 2, these requirements may need to be reviewed and a further risk assessment undertaken.

b) Documentation
Where risk assessment has shown that preparation by pharmacy / specialist aseptics is appropriate, standard operating procedures (SOPs) and worksheets specific to the ATMPs being used should be in place. These should include the activities detailed in Part A, Chapter 8. Worksheets specific to the gene therapy or cell therapy being prepared should record patient details and the appropriate details specified in Part A, Chapter 8.

c) Labelling

Labels should include the information specified in Part A, Chapter 8. If advanced therapy clinical trial products are classed as investigational medicinal products, they should be labelled as such.

Consideration should be given to the requirement for labelling transport containers with a biological hazard warning sign.

d) Training

It is essential that all staff involved in handling gene therapy vectors, or cellular and tissue products, are trained in the procedures specific to handling these therapies. Employees need to be aware of any risk associated with these therapies and to have an option not to be involved in the process. Staff handling these agents should not be pregnant, breastfeeding, or immunosuppressed. Staff training should be documented, recorded and regularly updated, as recommended in Part A, Chapter 9.

It is likely that in larger organisations who may be asked to prepare ATMPs there is a group of expert staff from a stem cell laboratory or from haematology who may be able to provide training in handling cells or may be able to perform the activity required with oversight from pharmacy.

e) Aseptic processing

Often advanced therapy products are of a very small volume and some require multiple dilutions to reconstitute them. The dilution process can be complex and calculations should be recorded and checked. Cellular and viral products are often quantified in units by the number of cells or viral particles that are present in 1ml. The measurement of volumes for dilution is critical to the dose the patient will receive, as doses in the region of 1×10^{12} viral particles or cells are not uncommon in a small volume of liquid. Sterile pyrogen-free micro pipettes may be considered instead of needles and syringes during preparation to increase accuracy. For the volume of liquid remaining in syringes and needles after administration, the dead volume compensation may be required in calculations and preparation. Systems should be designed in such a way that open procedures are not required. Training requirements should be considered prior to undertaking this type of preparation work.

f) Cleaning

Decontamination or cleaning procedures should be confirmed with individual suppliers. Particular care is required for advanced therapies as monitoring techniques do not validate the removal of viral material, and minimal exposure of GMOs to humans and the environment is required by the HSE. In such cases virucidal agents, which have proven activity against the gene therapy vectors involved, must be used. Cleaning processes should also ensure that any organic materials or proteins can be removed or denatured.

g) Storage

The majority of advanced therapy products require storage below -70°C. Storage facilities should be near the preparation area to minimise risk of spillage and contamination of other areas.

Freezers (-20° and -80°C) should be available for storage.

Cellular ATMPs are often cryopreserved and are often delivered at -80°C in an insulating storage vessel (dewar). Prolonged storage may require transfer to a liquid nitrogen tank. Training in the handling of liquid nitrogen will be required if pharmacy are involved in issuing these products, or an understanding of processes if providing oversight.

h) Transport

Gene therapies may be hazardous. Autologous cell therapies may not be hazardous but they are often the patient's individualised therapy, therefore they are not easily replaced (if at all); hence, transportation should be carefully planned.

Transport of GMOs within the hospital is subject to risk assessment. All transport outside of the hospital should comply with *The Carriage of Dangerous Goods by Road Regulations 1996*. It should be noted that work on the application of these regulations to gene therapy is ongoing, and it is likely that clinical products will be exempt. However all transport should be subject to risk assessment.

In practice if preparation for administration is to occur in a clinical area, it may be necessary to transport the product to the clinical area within its storage dewar, as shelf life post thaw is often as little as thirty minutes.

i) Waste disposal

Waste disposal procedures should be confirmed with individual suppliers. All waste should be sealed before removal from the isolator or safety cabinet.

Schedule 8 of *The Genetically Modified Organisms (Contained Use) Regulations 2014* makes reference to the availability of an autoclave on site or in the building. This guidance refers to equipment that is washed, sterilised and re-used. It should therefore be noted that, for the vast majority of products handled in pharmacy aseptic units, this will not apply as only sterile, single use disposable items are used (see Part A, Chapter 13).

All waste materials contaminated with GMOs should be inactivated, by autoclaving on site, incineration by a contractor licensed to handle GM waste, or by chemical inactivation. An audit trail should be in place.

j) Spillage

Spillage procedures are required and may have to be tailored to each product using information provided by the supplier. Procedures should "contain" any spilt gene therapy product and allow for its subsequent inactivation. The risk assessment and class of the GMO will determine the contents of "spillage kits". For example, a spillage kit may contain gloves, masks, aprons, goggles, disposable shoe covers, virucidal detergents, absorbent material, disposal forceps and a biohazard incineration bag. It is essential that spillage kits are available in areas where gene therapy is handled.

k) Administration

Every organisation should consider the training requirement for staff involved in the administration of cellular products. This is likely to be a post-qualification competency for nurses and an understanding of the specialist issues involved is advocated.

References

Directive 2001/18/EC of the European Parliament and of the Council of 12 March 2001 on the deliberate release into the environment of genetically modified organisms.

Directive 2001/83/EC of the European Parliament and of the Council of 6 November 2001 on the Community code relating to the manufacture of medicinal products.

Directive 2009/41/EC of the European Parliament and of the Council of 6 May 2009 on the contained use of genetically modified microorganisms.

European Commission (2015). *The Rules Governing Medicinal Products in the European Union. Volume 4 Good Manufacturing Practice Medicinal Products for Human and Veterinary Use. Annex 2: Manufacture of Biological Active Substances and Medicinal Products for Human Use.* Available at: **http://ec.europa.eu/health/files/eudralex/vol-4/ vol4-an22012-06_en.pdf** (accessed 19 May 2016).

Regulation (EC) No 1394/2007 of the European Parliament and the Council of 13 November 2007 on advanced therapy medicinal products and amending Directive 2001/83/EC and Regulation (EC) No 726/2004.

The Carriage of Dangerous Goods By Road Regulations 1996. SI 1996 No. 2095. London: The Stationery Office.

The Genetically Modified Organisms (Contained Use) Regulations 2014. SI 2014 No. 1663. London: The Stationery Office.

The Human Tissue (Quality and Safety for Human Application) Regulations 2007. SI 2007 No 1523. London: The Stationery Office.

The Medicines for Human Use (Clinical Trials) Regulations 2004. SI 2004 No.1031. London: The Stationery Office.

ACKNOWLEDGEMENTS

The Royal Pharmaceutical Society and NHS Pharmaceutical Quality Assurance Committee are grateful to the editor Dr Alison M Beaney, also to the individuals and organisations who have provided contributions and comment for the 5th edition of Quality Assurance of Aseptic Preparation Services: Standards. All the standards have been updated for this edition. The main contributors for this update are:

Richard Bateman	Quality Assurance Specialist Pharmacist East and South East England, Guy's and St Thomas' NHS Foundation Trust, UK
Alison M Beaney	Regional Quality Assurance Specialist North East and North Cumbria, Newcastle upon Tyne Hospitals NHS Foundation Trust, UK
Anne Black	Assistant Director of Pharmacy - Quality Assurance, Newcastle upon Tyne Hospitals NHS Foundation Trust, UK
Charlotte Gibb (on behalf of the NHS Pharmaceutical Aseptic Services Group)	Accountable Pharmacist, Pinderfields Hospital, The Mid Yorkshire Hospitals NHS Trust, UK
Joanne Hayes	Director of Technical Services, Stockport NHS Foundation Trust, UK
John Horncastle	Accountable Pharmacist, Newcastle upon Tyne Hospitals NHS Foundation Trust, UK
Mark Jackson	Director, Quality Control North West (Liverpool), UK
Paul Maltby (on behalf of the UK Radiopharmacy Group)	Formerly (now retired):- Principal Radiopharmacist, Royal Liverpool and Broadgreen University Hospitals, UK
Linda Musker (on behalf of the Microbiology Protocols Group)	Quality Assurance Specialist, Quality Control North West (Liverpool), NHS England North, UK
Mark Oldcorne (on behalf of the Microbiology Protocols Group)	All Wales QA Specialist Pharmacist, Betsi Cadwaladr University Health Board, Wrexham Maelor Hospital, NHS Wales, UK

John C Rhodes (on behalf of the Microbiology Protocols Group)	Quality Assurance Specialist, Stockton Quality Control Laboratory, North Tees & Hartlepool NHS Foundation Trust, UK
Mark Santillo (on behalf of the NHS National Research and Development Group)	Regional Quality Assurance Officer South West, Torbay and South Devon NHS Foundation Trust, UK
Karen Shield	Pharmacy Production Manager, Sunderland Royal Hospital, UK
Tim Sizer (on behalf of the Microbiology Protocols Group)	Regional Pharmaceutical Quality Assurance Pharmacist, NHS England South, UK
Lauren Stewart	Senior Pharmacist, Quality Assurance, Newcastle upon Tyne Hospitals NHS Foundation Trust, UK

With thanks to Leslie Rippon who provided valuable administrative assistance.

NHS Pharmaceutical Quality Assurance Committee Microbiology Protocols Group:

Sarah Hiom	All Wales Research and Development Pharmacist, NHS Wales, UK
Linda Musker	Quality Assurance Specialist, Quality Control North West (Liverpool), NHS England North, UK
Ayo Ogunsanlu	Pharmacy Executive Lead QA & QC and Q.P., Imperial College Healthcare NHS Trust, UK
Mark Oldcorne	All Wales QA Specialist Pharmacist, Betsi Cadwaladr University Health Board, Wrexham Maelor Hospital, NHS Wales, UK
Bernie Sanders	East Midlands Regional QA/QC Head NHS England Central, UK
Janet Shaw	Microbiology Laboratory Section Head; Quality Control North West (Liverpool), NHS England North, UK
Tim Sizer (Chair)	Regional Pharmaceutical Quality Assurance Pharmacist, NHS England South, UK

NHS Pharmaceutical Quality Assurance Committee Microbiology Protocols Group (continued):

Victoria Tickle	Lead Microbiologist, Stockton Quality Control Laboratory, North Tees & Hartlepool NHS Foundation Trust, UK
John C Rhodes	Quality Assurance Specialist, Stockton Quality Control Laboratory, North Tees & Hartlepool NHS Foundation Trust, UK

National NHS Pharmaceutical Research and Development Group:

Suresh Aiyalu	Principal Pharmacist, Aseptic Services Sandwell and West Birmingham Hospitals NHS Trust, UK
Andrew Barnes	Deputy Director of Pharmacy Quality Assurance Specialist Services East of England & Northamptonshire, UK
Wayne Goddard	Laboratory Manager, Stockton Quality Control Laboratory, North Tees & Hartlepool NHS Foundation Trust, UK
Mark Oldcorne	All Wales QA Specialist Pharmacist, Betsi Cadwaladr University Health Board, Wrexham Maelor Hospital, NHS Wales, UK
Mark Santillo (Chair)	Regional Quality Assurance Officer, Torbay & South Devon NHS Foundation Trust, UK
Phil Weir	Principal Scientist, Head of Scientific Services, Quality Control North West, Stockport, UK

Consultees

Consultees who responded included the following organisations:

Medicines and Healthcare products Regulatory Agency (MHRA)
NHS Pharmaceutical Quality Assurance Committee (PQAC)
Pharmaceutical Aseptic Services Group (PASG)
UK Radiopharmacy Group (UKRG)

The NHS Pharmaceutical Quality Assurance Committee, NHS Pharmaceutical Aseptic Services Group and UK Radiopharmacy Group include representatives from England, Scotland, Wales and Northern Ireland.

RPS Project Team:

Catherine Duggan	Director of Professional Development and Support
Sam Haddaway	Marketing Executive
Julia Kettlewell	Head of Marketing
Rachel Norton	Senior Professional Support Pharmacist
Parita Patel	Product Manager, RPS Publishing
Harvinder Sondh	Director of Marketing and Product Development, RPS Publishing
Ruth Wakeman	Assistant Director of Professional Development and Support

With thanks to colleagues in RPS Publishing, RPS Finance and Resources, and RPS website team for their valuable assistance.

ACKNOWLEDGEMENTS

INDEX

A

INDEX

S

NOTES

QUALITY ASSURANCE OF ASEPTIC PREPARATION SERVICES:
STANDARDS HANDBOOK PARTS A&B